good clean beauty

Over **100** Natural Recipes
for a Glowing, Beautiful You

CAROLINE BERCAW · ISABEL BERCAW

ROCK
POINT
QUARTOKNOWS.COM
NEW YORK, NY

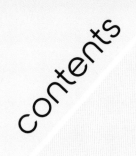

contents

INTRODUCTION

Let's face it: Keeping ourselves looking gorgeous can get pricey. Between hair, makeup, and body care needs, one trip to the mall for all those lotions and potions can drain a person's bank account quicker than you can say "Spa me!"

And then there's the issue of ingredients. Commercially manufactured beauty products often have dozens of unpronounceable ingredients that sound as if they came directly from Dr. Strange's lab. What's a health- and budget-conscious Glamazon to do?! Scale back on personal care? (Never!) If you're like us, grooming is not only a necessity, it's a lifelong obsession.

So, several years ago, when we realized we could make our own beauty products naturally, at home, it was as if a glitter bomb of excitement went off in our heads. Since then, we've been experimenting with everything from eye shadow to highlighter, blush to conditioning treatments. And, if you're willing to follow along with us, we're ready to teach you everything you need to know to make your very own, utterly exciting, nontoxic, totally customized beauty arsenal!

The best part about the recipes in this book is that you don't have to be an expert to make them. They're surprisingly easy, even for a DIY newbie. And, in many cases, you might have most of the ingredients already sitting in your pantry. (Any missing

ingredients can be easily ordered online). Before you know it, you'll be confidently concocting hair masks, shampoos, bronzers, blush, and maybe even deodorant!

But before we dive into the good stuff, here's a little background info: We've been superfans of natural DIY bath and beauty for practically as long as we could open a jar of organic coconut oil. When we were just ten and twelve years old, we started making bath bombs, body scrubs, lip balm, and eye shadow in our basement as a hobby. Our friends and family liked our creations so much that we soon found ourselves selling our most popular product (bath bombs) at pop-up shopping events in our community. And finally, in April of 2015, at the ripe old ages of twelve and fourteen, we officially co-founded our bath and body products company, Da Bomb® Bath.

Fast-forward to today. Our fun little pastime has somehow grown into a multimillion-dollar company! We now sell to more than 25,000 stores all over the United States. Though we've expanded our product line to include a full range of products like exfoliating scrubs, therapeutic bath salts, foaming bath powder, and lip gloss, our commitment to simple ingredients remains very much at the top of our minds. And no matter how busy it gets in our test kitchen, we're usually there developing new recipes for commercial *and* at-home use. When we formulate new

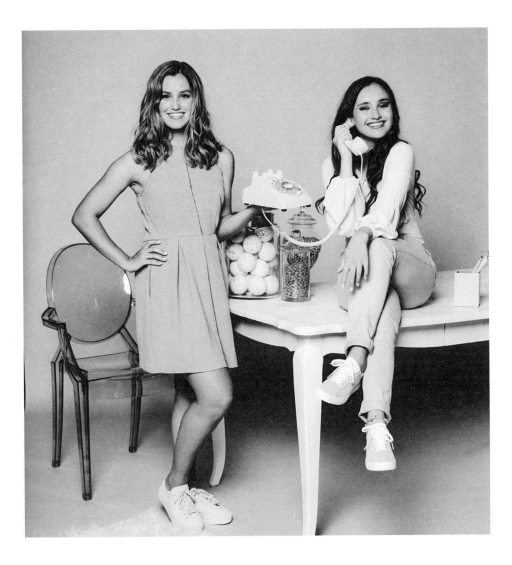

recipes for commercial sale, a product needs to go through lots of testing to make sure it meets all the rules and regulations and has a retail-ready shelf life. But when you make something at home for immediate use, you have a whole new level of freedom to minimize ingredients and maximize freshness.

So whether you're ready to devote an entire wing of your home to natural makeup and body care or you're hoping to start by investing in just a few key ingredients, we'll have you flexing your beauty formulation muscles in no time! Are you ready to begin? Then head over to your kitchen and let's get this party started!

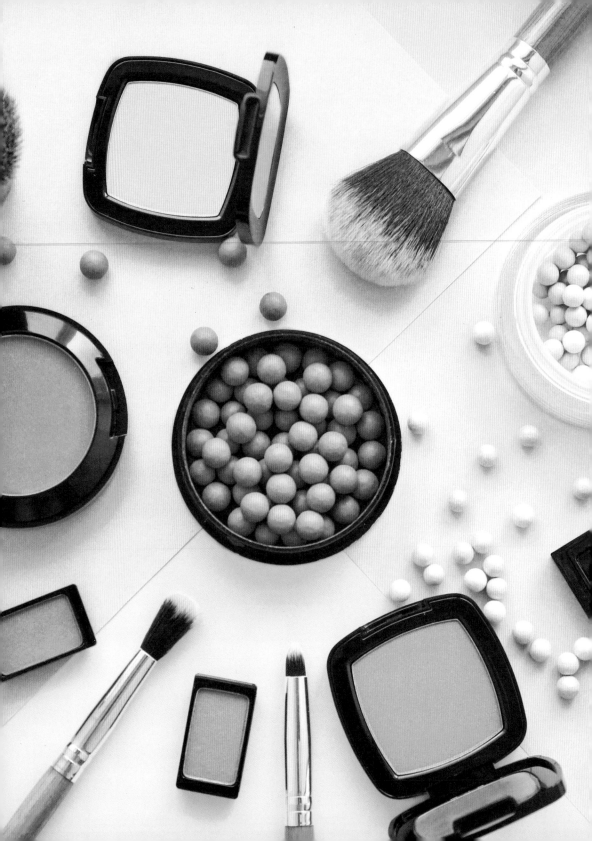

ingredients
+
benefits

————

MAKING YOUR OWN NATURAL MAKEUP, HAIR CARE, SKIN CARE,
AND BEAUTY PRODUCTS IS ALREADY SO MUCH FUN. TO KNOW
THAT THESE BEAUTY PRODUCTS HAVE ADDED BENEFITS IS
A HUGE BONUS. WHAT FOLLOWS IS A LIST OF ALL-NATURAL
INGREDIENTS THAT ARE USED IN THE RECIPES IN THIS BOOK AND
ALL OF THE INCREDIBLE WAYS THAT THEY BENEFIT YOU—
IN ADDITION TO MAKING YOU FEEL BEAUTIFUL.

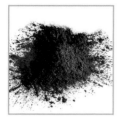

activated charcoal
Effective at removing toxins from the skin. Can effectively treat and prevent breakouts.

almond oil Keeps the skin and hair hydrated by preventing water loss. This antiaging, vitamin E–laden oil protects against sun damage and is a wonderful choice for those with sensitive skin.

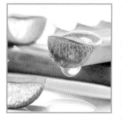

aloe vera gel
This antioxidant-filled gel has exfoliating enzymes that help smooth the skin. It has known antiaging benefits; it prevents fine lines from deepening. This gel is anti-inflammatory and is beneficial for those with dry skin or acne.

apple cider vinegar This vinegar has two components that help with a healthy complexion: acetic acid and citric acid. Acetic acid can help treat acne and eczema because of its antimicrobial and antifungal properties. Citric acid is an alpha hydroxy acid that can slow the aging process by decreasing wrinkles.

argan oil This Moroccan oil is from the pit of the argan tree fruit. It is rich in oleic and linoleic acids, otherwise known as omega-6s. This oil is rich in vitamin E and healthy fats, making it beneficial for healthy skin and hair. There are so many antioxidant-helping compounds in this special oil—CoQ10 and melatonin are two notable players. Argan oil helps decrease inflammation when applied to the skin and it also increases skin elasticity.

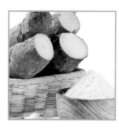

arrowroot powder
This gluten-free powder has been used in society for more than 7,000 years. It is from the roots of the Marantaceae family of plants. This starch is used in cosmetics and has been shown to help cure blemishes. Its sweat-absorbing capabilities also make it a great addition to deodorant. This moisture-wicking ability makes it a go-to choice for including in dry shampoo.

avocado This antioxidant-stuffed superfood plumps skin because of its high concentration of healthy fats. This creamy fruit is also packed full of antiaging antioxidants.

avocado oil This oil has the power to neutralize free radicals and can speed healing because of the fatty acids it contains. This makes it a great oil for quickly healing a mark left by acne.

baking soda This alkaline powder can fight bacteria and soothe inflammation, making it a natural go-to for skin care when fighting acne. This substance is a wonderful exfoliant, as it naturally removes dead skin cells.

banana This vitamin-packed fruit is full of skin-soothing benefits. Vitamin C helps produce collagen and controls oil production, while lectin helps ward off acne-causing bacteria. This fruit is known for its high potassium content, which helps the skin retain moisture.

basil oil This oil comes from sweet basil, a plant that is a part of the mint family. Its spicy and inviting scent also contains loads of antioxidants and has the ability to dispel odor-causing bacteria.

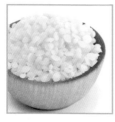

beeswax pellets This wax is a combination of pollen and plant wax. The natural ability of beeswax to stay in place makes it an ideal ingredient in cosmetics. Beeswax also falls smoothly against the skin while allowing the skin to breathe. This hydrating wax helps lock moisture into the skin. They come in white and different shades of beige, and can even be a little brown or honey-colored. **Note:** When white is needed, it is noted in the recipes.

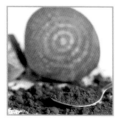

beetroot powder Beetroot increases blood circulation, is full of vitamin C, and has both potassium and antioxidants as part of its health portfolio. Beetroot can exfoliate dead cells and has a lovely color that is perfectly suited to cosmetics.

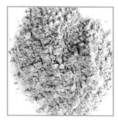

bentonite clay This is nature's magnet: It pulls impurities out of the skin, including excess oils. It also replenishes the skin with essential minerals like magnesium, calcium, and silicone. The gentle exfoliating properties of this clay combined with its acne-abolishing properties make it a blemish buster.

bergamot oil This citrusy oil is from the rind of the fruit found on the Southeast Asian–derived bergamot orange tree. It is a soothing antibacterial oil and an effective anti-inflammatory acne treatment.

calamine lotion This blend of zinc oxide and ferric oxide has been used by human beings for thousands of years. It can effectively treat acne, soften skin, lighten dark spots, minimize scars, and serve as a moisturizer and sunscreen.

cane sugar This sugar's naturally occurring glycolic acid promotes skin cell turnover and gets rid of oil and other skin-clogging matter. These properties make cane sugar the perfect ingredient in scrubs, exfoliants, soaks, and face masks.

carrot seed oil This oil has sun protection properties, as it carries a natural SPF. This oil also has polyphenols, which are antioxidants that protect against free radical damage. It can protect hair and skin from external damage from environmental pollutants because of its high level of antioxidants.

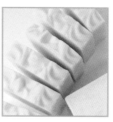

castile soap Though traditionally made with olive oil from the Mediterranean, this natural vegetable-based soap can be made from a variety of oils. This soap is gentle on the skin yet strong enough to fight bacteria.

castor oil This oil comes from extracting and heating the oil from castor beans. A fatty acid called ricinoleic acid is prevalent in castor oil. This monosaturated fatty acid helps keep the skin hydrated. This makes the oil a natural selection for hair care, body oils, and cosmetics.

chamomile oil This multipurpose oil comes from the petals of the chamomile flower. It has been found to relieve depression and reduce anger, and it can lessen the appearance of scars on the skin.

cinnamon This sweet-smelling, warm brown powder can naturally bring blood and, with it, nutrients to the surface of the skin. This causes a natural plumping, which can be lovely when applied to the lips. Cinnamon can also be used to help stimulate hair growth and cleanse the scalp.

cocoa powder This chocolaty powder comes from ground cocoa beans that have had the cocoa butter separated from them. Antioxidants in cocoa powder are naturally antiaging and acne-fighting. This rich brown powder has also been shown to increase blood flow to the skin's surface, creating a tightening effect.

coconut milk All of the nutrients in this liquid that comes from the meat of a mature coconut make it the perfect choice to help keep hair healthy and strong. The creamy liquid contains enough vitamin C to help combat the fine lines and discoloration associated with aging. It's also super hydrating and can help with dry skin.

coconut oil Coconut oil contains more than eight medium-chain fatty acids that make up more than 65 percent of its composition. Coconut oil goes from solid to liquid form quickly, remaining solid at room temperature but melting quickly when coming into contact with the skin. The lauric acid in coconut oil can kill the bacteria that cause acne. As an added bonus, this oil is super hydrating and can be used on skin, in hair, and in cosmetics.

coconut water Coconut water is the juice that comes from green coconuts. This water contains age-fighting cytokines that help generate new cell growth. It is hydrating and pH balancing, making it a natural fit for skin care products. The vitamin K helps promote healthy hair that stays strong.

coffee The caffeine content in coffee helps increase blood flow to the skin when applied topically. This can help with circulation and decrease the appearance of cellulite. Coffee is also effective at combating inflammation because of its chlorogenic acid, which helps decrease puffiness in the face.

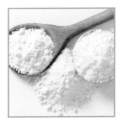

cornstarch Cornstarch is a natural moisture absorber, which makes it a fantastic addition to deodorant, dry shampoo, and cosmetic setting powders.

egg whites Egg whites are virtually pure protein. It is commonly believed that this protein can help control or minimize oil production in the skin and can temporarily tighten the skin.

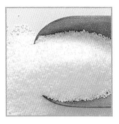

epsom salt (also known as magnesium sulfate) This pure mineral compound has many natural beauty benefits. It is a gentle exfoliant and doubles as a stress reliever and pain reducer when added to a bath. It is also believed to have detoxifying properties.

eucalyptus oil This oil comes from the eucalyptus tree's silvery green leaves. It has many benefits due to its antimicrobial properties. It can help you breathe more easily and works as a disinfectant, assists mental clarity, treats acne, and stimulates your immunity.

frankincense oil This spicy, earthy, warm oil is derived from the resin of the Boswellia tree, which is native to Africa and the Middle East. The oil is believed to have antiaging properties and to be effective in treating fine lines.

grapefruit oil This mood-brightening oil that comes from the peel of a grapefruit smells delicious and has further benefits. In addition to lifting your spirits (it is believed to help combat depression), this oil can help with fatigue and acne due to its antibacterial and antifungal properties.

grapeseed oil This oil comes from the grape seeds that remain after making wine. Its high concentration of omega-6 fatty acids and vitamin E makes it an ideal addition to your beauty routine. These components help protect the skin from toxins in the environment while providing a deep level of moisture.

hibiscus powder This powder from the hibiscus flower has the ability to block elastase, an enzyme that breaks down elastin in the skin. Elastin is what keeps the skin looking tight and youthful. This antioxidant-rich powder also assists with balancing hyperpigmentation and smoothing skin with gentle acids that have a mild exfoliating effect.

honey The antibacterial properties of honey combined with its deeply hydrating effects make it a natural fit for beauty products. This sweet treat works wonders in face masks and hair masks.

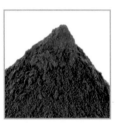

iron oxides These are simply the combination of the compounds of iron and oxygen, and have been used in cosmetics since the early 1900s. They are used to color or tint the cosmetic. Iron oxides come in a variety of nontoxic natural colors, allowing a DIYer to have creative flexibility and safety.

jasmine oil The beautiful and fragrant white flowers of the jasmine plant are the source of this syrupy, sweet-smelling oil. This oil is thought to be mood-boosting, increasing feelings of energy and romance. It is a multilayered oil, having the properties of an antiseptic and an aphrodisiac. This oil is also used to treat inflammation.

jojoba oil This oil comes from the nut of the jojoba plant, a North American native that can survive the harshest conditions. This oil does a wonderful job of holding hydration in the skin and can fight all kinds of bacteria and fungi. The natural vitamin E in this oil fights free radical damage and doesn't clog pores. It is also thought to aid in collagen production.

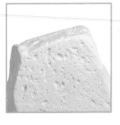

kaolin clay This is a silica-based clay, which means it is great at absorbing oils without reducing the moisture in your skin. It is a gentle exfoliant that is also simultaneously hydrating. Kaolin clay is commonly used in cosmetics and face masks for its skin-soothing properties.

kukui oil This oil comes from the nut of Hawaii's state tree: the candlenut or kukui nut tree. This oil is packed with healthy fats, antioxidants, and vitamins C, D, and E. The linoleic and linolenic fatty acids that are present in this oil make it perfect for use in hair-strengthening products. The hydrating qualities of this oil can help prevent hair from breaking. This powerful oil also helps with antiaging, as it provides deeply penetrating hydration to the skin.

lavender oil This calming oil, traditionally used to assist with stress reduction and sleep, is from the purple lavender plant. It has powerful antibacterial properties, making it a perfect inclusion in any skin care or hair care product, specifically those used before it's time to unwind for the night. This oil is also a powerful acne buster, as it hydrates and eradicates bacteria before it enters the pores.

lemon juice This alkaline citrus juice from the bright-yellow lemon helps balance pH levels and battle acne. It is also touted as a blackhead treatment and helps with discoloration of the skin. The citric acid in lemon juice helps turn over skin cells because it is a natural alpha hydroxy acid. The vitamin C in the juice helps brighten the skin because it can increase collagen production while blocking skin from harmful pollutants.

lemon oil This oil comes from pressing the peel of a lemon. It has been shown to be energizing and to battle stress, combat acne, and reduce anxiety.

macadamia oil This oil comes from the nutrient-loaded macadamia nut. Its high concentration of fatty acids, specifically palmitoleic acid, helps heal the skin, slows the aging process (it's firming!), and moisturizes. This oil is ideal for use on the skin because it absorbs quickly and doesn't leave behind a sticky feeling.

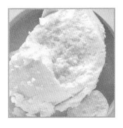

mango butter This creamy butter comes from the seed of a mango. This butter is chock-full of antioxidants, which makes it amazing at reducing inflammation and slowing the aging process. Mango butter hydrates and protects against UV radiation. **Note:** When working with mango butter, you need to ensure that it goes from hot to cold quickly so that it doesn't get grainy. Immediately after mixing all of the ingredients, put the mixture in the freezer to make sure that it stays smooth.

mica powder

This beautifully shimmery mineral comes in a variety of colors and shades and adds sparkle to beauty products. This organic substance is generally considered safe for all skin types. Mica powder is perfect when you want to add a bit of glitter to any product.

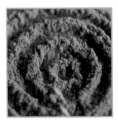

morrocan lava clay / ghassoul clay

This volcanic clay goes by many names: ghassoul clay, rhassoul clay, oxide clay, and red clay. It works magic on skin because its negatively charged properties pull positively charged toxins out of pores. This deep clean is also hydrating, so you can safely use it on the hair as well as the skin.

olive oil

This antioxidant-laden oil helps fight UV rays, staves off aging, and is incredibly hydrating. It also touts antibacterial benefits. This oil is versatile and can be used all over the body and hair.

patchouli oil

This oil has a powerful and distinct smell that many people find pleasing. It is earthy, warm, spicy, and a bit sweet. This scent is thought to reduce depression and stress, and it's also an acne fighter and beautiful addition to a perfume.

peppermint oil

This brightly scented oil is believed to increase energy levels and lift the mood. It is also antibacterial, which is an added skin-saving benefit. Additionally, this oil has anti-inflammatory and skin-toning effects.

pomegranate oil

This skin-beneficial oil from the seeds of the pomegranate nourishes the skin with linoleic acid, vitamin C, and punicic acid. Fatty acids and antioxidants help combat signs of aging. This oil can also fight acne and inflammation.

raspberry seed oil

This fruit oil is the perfect addition to face creams, serums, and other cosmetics because it is beneficial for the skin. It contains antioxidants and has hydrating properties, so it can assist with skin suppleness and combat aging, specifically because of its ellagic acid, which decreases collagen loss. This oil also provides sun protection.

rose oil

This oil is thought to sharpen memory, elevate the mood, and soften the skin. It has a powerfully fragrant scent, which makes it an ideal addition to any beauty product if you want an olfactory boost.

rose water

This floral water comes from steaming rose petals. This delightful water reduces redness because it has many anti-inflammatory properties. In addition to its skin-soothing abilities, the scent from this water has been shown to have positive effects on mood, decreasing feelings of depression and anxiety.

rosehip oil Though the name may lead you to believe that this comes from a rose, it actually comes from the seeds of the wild rosehip fruit. It is full of fatty acids and carotenoids (a form of antioxidants). This allows the skin to be protected from free radical damage and stay hydrated. This oil also has a high vitamin C content, which makes it a powerful tool in combating aging.

rosemary oil This oil is thought to increase memory, reduce stress, and increase hair growth. It is a lovely aromatic to add to beauty blends.

sandalwood oil This oil has a musky scent that is a grounding addition to any fragrance or beauty oil. Sandalwood is believed to have many aromatherapy benefits, such as improving sleep, reducing anxiety, and increasing mental alertness.

sea salt The texture of sea salt makes it a perfect exfoliator. Its detoxifying benefits also make it a natural fit for a bath soak.

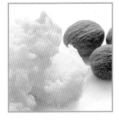

shea butter This vitamin A–packed creamy butter derived from the nuts of the shea tree has been found to increase collagen production, has anti-inflammatory and antiaging properties, and immediately improves the softness of skin. This butter is also full of skin-loving vitamin E and lots of fatty acids. It is also thought to combat cellulite. **Note:** When working with shea butter, you need to ensure that it goes from hot to cold quickly so that it

doesn't get grainy. Immediately after mixing all of the ingredients, put the mixture in the freezer to make sure that it stays smooth.

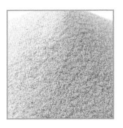

silica This naturally occurring mineral absorbs moisture, making it a natural fit for a setting powder, a dry shampoo, or an antiperspirant. It also provides a smooth texture to cosmetics.

spirulina This deep-green algae powder provides a wonderful way to naturally add color to cosmetics. It also contains antiaging vitamin E and has the ability to tone the skin.

strawberries This vitamin A– and vitamin C–packed fruit has many skin benefits. The naturally occurring salicylic acid can fight blackheads. This fruit can also diminish discoloration, fight acne, has antiaging properties, and can combat dark circles.

tea tree oil This inedible oil has strong anti-inflammatory and antibacterial components, making it an obvious choice when selecting a treatment for acne.

vanilla extract An unexpected source of free radical protection due to its antioxidant content, vanilla can also decrease inflammation and fight depression.

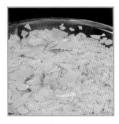

vegetable emulsifying wax

Oil and water don't work well together and that is where this wax comes in handy. This wax binds them together so that water and oil can cooperate in creating beauty products. This wax also affects the creaminess of a product.

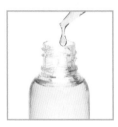

vegetable glycerin

This translucent liquid usually comes from palm, soybean, or coconut oils. It is highly emulsifying and improves the condition of the skin. This hydrating substance can also provide a barrier to protect the skin. These qualities make it a popular addition to cosmetics and skin care.

vitamin E oil Vitamin E is an important antioxidant. It is easily absorbed when used topically and is a great hydrator for very dry or sensitive skin. This makes vitamin E oil a good ingredient to add to moisturizers and eye treatments.

witch hazel One of this liquid's strong suits is decreasing inflammation through its powerful anti-inflammatory properties like tannins and gallic acid. This makes it a great choice for shrinking pores with skin toners or fighting acne with a facial cleanser.

ylang ylang oil The aroma of this oil from the flowers of the ylang ylang tree is relaxing and works as an antidepressant. This oil's scent makes it a good choice for perfumes and deodorants. It also helps combat blemishes and strengthen the hair.

yogurt The natural alpha hydroxy acid found in yogurt in the form of lactic acid helps with skin cell turnover and reduces the appearance of aging. The antifungal component of yogurt makes it a great acne treatment. It is also super hydrating and works beautifully in a hair mask.

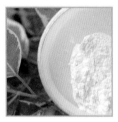

zinc oxide

This substance is an incredible acne treatment and an ideal sunblock. Zinc oxide also keeps skin hydrated, lowers inflammation, and is antiaging.

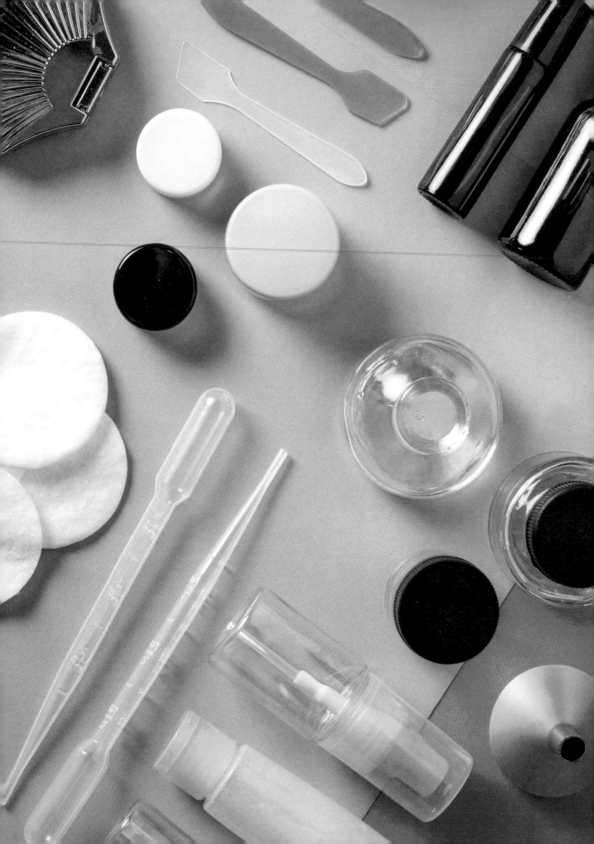

supplies
+
equipment

———

ONE OF THE MOST EXCITING STEPS IN BECOMING A DIY BEAUTY EXPERT IS TRACKING DOWN BEAUTIFUL VESSELS TO HOLD YOUR CREATIONS. THESE CAN BE PURCHASED ONLINE, OR EVEN REPURPOSED USING CONTAINERS YOU ALREADY OWN! WE LIKE TO USE GLASS VESSELS WHENEVER POSSIBLE, BUT ANY SIMILAR VESSEL WILL WORK. THERE'S PLENTY OF INSPIRATION IN THE PAGES THAT FOLLOW, ALONG WITH A LIST OF SUPPLIES YOU MIGHT WANT TO KEEP ON HAND.

blender Used to quickly incorporate and blend ingredients.

coffee maker Used to brew coffee to include in a recipe.

cosmetic compacts These can be used to hold pressed powders, bronzers, and foundations.

cotton rounds These work as an absorbent item that hold homemade makeup remover.

double boiler This instrument melts oils, fats, and solids into a purely liquid state. Don't have a double boiler? Not a problem. Use an 8 ounce (240-milileter) glass jar with lid instead. Put all the ingredients that would be placed in the double boiler into a glass jar and place the glass jar into a pot, then add water to come halfway up the sides of the glass jar. Let this water get hot and melt the ingredients directly in the glass jar. If it's hard to stir the ingredients inside the jar, use a chopstick. **Note:** In addition, for safety reasons, we recommend using glass vessels for all recipes that require heating, since plastic containers run the risk of melting. However, if you do decide to use plastic in these recipes, be sure the mixture isn't too hot when poured into the plastic vessel.

dust mask Use this to protect against breathing in fine particles when working with mica powder and dust-like powders.

foam dispenser (8 oz /240 ml) This dispenser is used to distribute foaming homemade cleansers.

freezer You will need access to a small amount of freezer space to help some of the recipes cool quickly.

funnels (small and medium) These are helpful when transferring mixtures from a double boiler or a mixing bowl to a container.

glass bottle with dropper lid (4 oz / 120 ml) This size bottle is ideal for distributing serums, hair treatments, and body oils.

glass bottle with dropper lid (1 oz / 30 ml) This size bottle is ideal for holding highly concentrated products like liquid highlighter.

glass bottle with pump top (16 oz / 480 ml) This type of container is perfect for holding shampoo, conditioner, and bodywash. It is also a useful size for dispensing lotions.

glass bottle with spray top (4oz / 120 ml) The ideal size bottle for dispensing toner.

glass cosmetic containers with lid (3 ml) These small containers are a wonderful size for eye shadows (both powder and cream).

Note About Vessels: We prefer to use glass vessels whenever possible, and all the recipes in this book were made with glass vessels. However, there are all kinds of vessels to choose from. If you chose to use plastic, be sure they are BPA free.

glass cosmetic container with sifter and lid (50 g) The perfect size for lip balm, solid highlighters, powder mineral makeup, and a variety of other applications.

glass jar with lid (8 oz / 240 ml) If you don't have a double boiler, an 8-ounce (240-milileter) glass jar—a mason jar works well—can serve as a replacement when paired with hot water and a saucepan. (See "Double Boiler" opposite for instructions.)

glass lip gloss container with brush tip applicator (10 ml) This container is the right size to throw in your purse or makeup bag.

glass mascara tube with wand (10 ml) This tube holds homemade mascara.

glass roll-on bottle (15 ml) This is the ideal bottle for transporting fragrance and rollable essential oil.

glass spray bottle (4 oz / 120 ml) This bottle is used to hold a variety of setting sprays.

glass spray bottle (16 oz / 480 ml) This bottle is used to hold a variety of hair sprays.

ice tray This is used to freeze liquid items.

measuring cups You will use a standard set of measuring cups frequently when creating the recipes.

measuring spoons You will use a standard set of measuring spoons frequently when creating the recipes.

mixing bowls Small- and medium-size mixing bowls are used for combining ingredients.

mixing fork This is used to smash and incorporate ingredients.

mixing spoons A mixing spoon can be used to stir ingredients together so that they become fully incorporated.

mixing stick or chopstick When stirring a substance in a narrow container, a thin mixing stick—or chopstick—works well.

parchment paper This keeps things from sticking to a surface.

pipettes These can be used to transfer a small amount of material into a tiny opening and are especially helpful when working with mascara and lip gloss containers.

saucepan This can be used to heat liquid so that ingredients can melt and incorporate.

silicone squeeze bottles (3 oz / 90 ml) These bottles hold slightly viscous concoctions like facial primers.

tamping tool This is used to press down a powdery substance so that it is compact. It is helpful when pressing makeup into a cosmetic compact (an espresso tamper works especially well).

whisk This handy tool works well for blending, whipping, and stirring ingredients together.

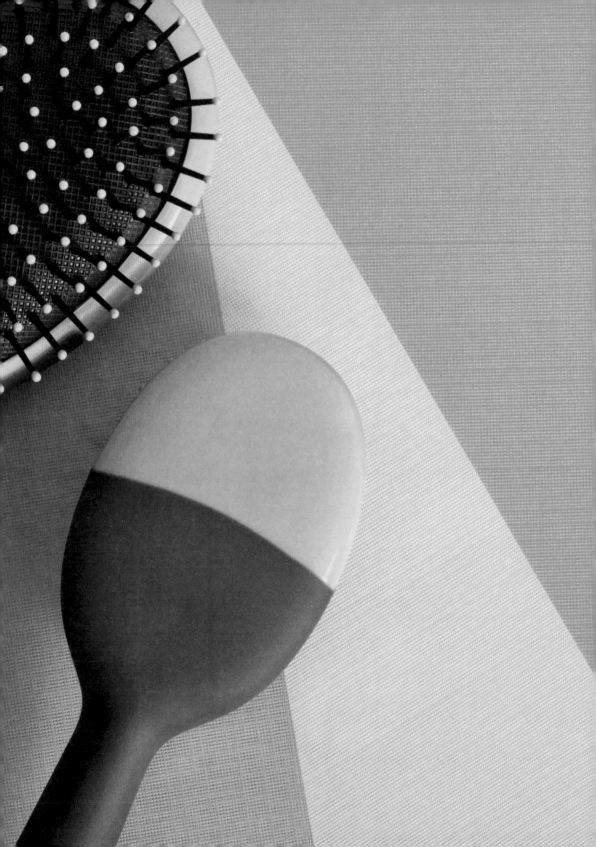

HAIR

Hold on to your tresses, people—this is going to be fun! (And moisturizing.) When it comes to feeling confident in yourself, nothing beats clean, healthy locks. In addition to regular trims and a bit of brushing or combing, a little extra effort can pay off in a big way. This section is chock-full of everything from shine-enhancing mists to sprays and deep-conditioning masks, as well as wonderful options for washing and hydrating. Whether you're known for having flowing locks, a glorious Afro, sleek braids, a chic crop, or a mop top, we'll have you looking your best in no time!

genie in a bottle hair spray

Wouldn't it be great to find something in a bottle that would grant you a good hair day? If this seems like a wish that's out of reach, consider this spray your own personal genie. The magic is in the perfect combination of hydration, a transcendent scent, and just the right amount of shimmer.

what you will need

- **16-oz (480-ml) glass spray bottle**
- **Funnel**
- **30 drops jasmine oil**

- **2 tsp mica powder (gold)**
- **2 cups (480 ml) distilled water**
- **1 tbsp (15 ml) aloe vera gel (clear)**

MAKES ONE 16-OUNCE (480-ML) BOTTLE

HAIR

step by step

1. Put the jasmine oil and mica powder in the spray bottle.

2. Heat the water in a pot on the stovetop until hot.

3. Take the water off the heat and add the aloe vera gel. Stir until dissolved.

4. Wait for the water to cool from hot to warm. Use a funnel to pour the mixture into the bottle and carefully add the top.

5. Shake well until all of the oil is incorporated into the warm liquid.

6. Let cool before spraying onto hair.*

how to use Spray all over hair for subtle shimmer and shine.

tip Turn a quick hairstyle into something special. On those days when you only have time to throw your hair into a ponytail, take an extra moment to shake up a bottle of this and give your ponytail a spritz. Subtle sparkle takes you from blah to babe.

modification Looking for some extra shine? Double the amount of mica powder. Want to switch up your look? Use different color mica powders for a totally different experience. Try hot pink for those days when you have a wild streak. Use an iridescent mica for a unicorn effect. Throw in a mica powder that matches your hair for a subtle shimmer. The combinations are endless.

* It is natural for the ingredients to separate. Shake well to fully combine all the ingredients before spraying.

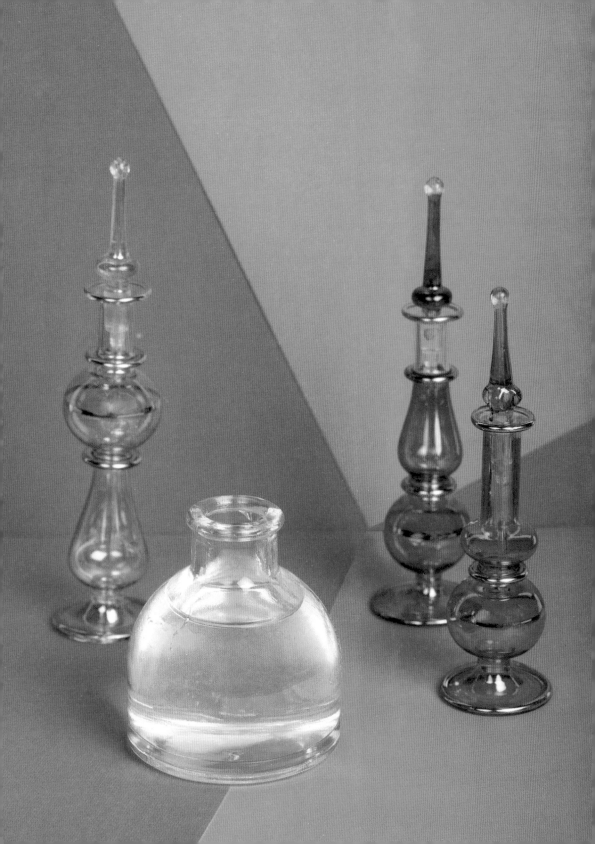

feelin' salty hair spray

If you're feeling salty about not being close to a beach, don't fret!

what you will need

- 16-oz (480-ml) glass spray bottle
- Funnel
- 1 tsp sea salt
- 1 tsp magnesium sulfate (Epsom salt)
- 1 tsp almond oil
- 1 tsp jojoba oil
- 30 drops coconut essential oil
- 2 cups (480 ml) distilled water
- 1 tbsp (15 ml) aloe vera gel (clear)

MAKES ONE 16-OUNCE (480-ML) BOTTLE

step by step

1. Put the sea salt, magnesium sulfate, and oils in the spray bottle.

2. Heat the water on the stovetop until the water is hot.

3. Take the water off the heat and add the aloe vera gel. Stir until dissolved.

4. Wait for the water to cool from hot to warm. Use a funnel to pour the mixture into the bottle and carefully add the top.

5. Shake well until all the salt and oil are incorporated into the liquid.

6. Let cool before spraying onto hair.*

how to use Spray all over hair and let air dry for a naturally textured look. Spray and scrunch hair if you want wilder waves.

* It is natural for the ingredients to separate. Shake well to fully combine all the ingredients before spraying.

beautiful summer hair mist

This is perfect for hair that looks glossy, feels soft, and smells as if you are walking through a rose garden.

what you will need

- 16-oz (480-ml) glass spray bottle
- Funnel
- 20 drops rose oil
- 1 tbsp (15 ml) jojoba oil
- 1 tbsp (15 ml) almond oil
- 2 cups (480 ml) distilled water
- 1 tbsp (15 ml) vegetable glycerin

MAKES ONE 16-OUNCE (480-ML) BOTTLE

step by step

1. Put the oils in the spray bottle.

2. Heat the water in pot on the stovetop until hot.

3. Take the water off the heat and add the vegetable glycerin. Stir until fully incorporated.

4. Wait for the water to cool from hot to warm. Use a funnel to pour the mixture into the bottle and carefully add the top.

5. Shake well until all the ingredients are incorporated.

6. Let cool before spraying onto hair.*

how to use Spray all over hair for shine and fragrance.

* It is natural for the ingredients to separate. Shake well to fully combine all the ingredients before spraying.

hydration station hair mist

If your hair looks like the embodiment of the Sahara Desert you need to keep your hair hydrated. For a mist that locks in moisture, increases shine, and smells light and fresh, try this magic mist.

what you will need

- 16-oz (480-ml) glass spray bottle
- Funnel
- 2 tsp olive oil
- 2 tsp almond oil

- 20 drops rose oil
- 1 cup (240 ml) rose water
- 1 cup (240 ml) distilled water
- 1 tbsp (15 ml) aloe vera gel

MAKES ONE 16-OUNCE (480-ML) BOTTLE

step by step

1. Put the olive oil, almond oil, rose oil, and rose water in the spray bottle.

2. Heat the water in a pot on the stovetop until hot.

3. Take the water off the heat and add the aloe vera gel. Stir until incorporated.

4. Wait for the water to cool from hot to warm. Use a funnel to pour the mixture into the bottle and carefully add the top.

5. Shake well before use.*

how to use Spray all over hair for a layer of hydration. Reapply as needed.

tip You can also spray this on wet hair to double as a leave-in conditioner and hair detangler.

modification For a lighter, beachier option, you can substitute fractionated coconut oil for the olive oil and any tropical scented oil for the rose oil.

It is natural for the ingredients to separate. Shake well to fully combine all the ingredients before spraying.

sunray highlighter spritz

Highlights can quickly brighten up your look. Trying to get the most natural highlights possible? Use the sun. To help boost the sun's incredible hair-brightening abilities, this spray uses fresh lemon juice to speed the time needed to get those natural highlights. Take this with you on vacation, to the beach, or just spray it in your hair before spending some much-needed time outside soaking up your vitamin D.

what you will need

- 16-oz (480-ml) spray bottle
- Funnel
- 6 tbsp (90 ml) lemon juice
- 30 drops grapefruit essential oil
- 2 cups (480 ml) distilled water

MAKES ONE 16-OUNCE (480-ML) BOTTLE

HAIR

step by step

1. Use a funnel to pour the lemon juice and essential oil into the spray bottle.

2. Use a funnel to pour the water into the spray bottle until it is filled to the top. Discard any extra water.

3. Shake well.

4. Store in the refrigerator.*

how to use Spray liberally on hair and comb through to make sure that the spray is evenly incorporated. Feel free to reapply throughout your time in the sun.

tip Having this spray in the fridge preserves the life of the lemon juice and gives you a quick and cool pick-me-up on a sunny day. Want to keep your cool all day long? Keep this lightening spray in your cooler at the beach. A quick mist will refresh you and brighten your locks.

modification If you want to be able to store this concoction unrefrigerated for a while, just add a few drops of vodka. It works as a natural preservative! You can also add a little sea salt to this spray to make it do double duty—it will help lighten your strands and give you beachy waves.

It is natural for the ingredients to separate. Shake well to fully combine all the ingredients before spraying.

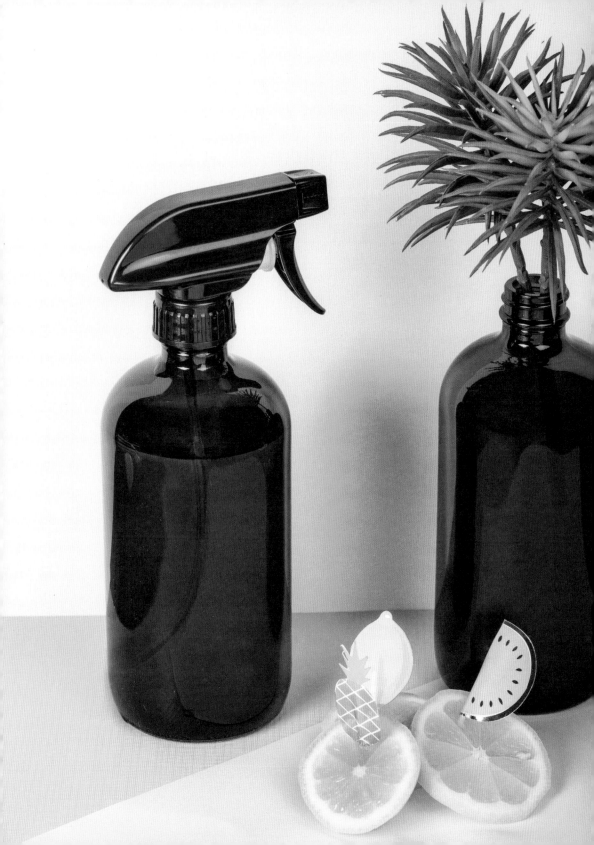

sunken treasure sea spray

Want loose beach waves and texture? The salt and oils combine for a mixture that is both volumizing and hydrating. The addition of mica powder adds a subtle shimmer.

what you will need

- 16-oz (480-ml) glass spray bottle
- Funnel
- ½ tsp mica powder (color of your choice)
- 1 cup (240 ml) rose water

- 2 tsp fractionated coconut oil
- 1 tbsp (15 ml) Epsom salt
- 1 cup (240 ml) distilled water

MAKES ONE 16-OUNCE (480-ML) BOTTLE

step by step

1. Put the mica powder, rose water, fractionated coconut oil, and Epsom salt in the spray bottle.

2. Heat the water in a pot on the stove until hot.

3. Use a funnel to carefully transfer the hot water to the spray bottle and carefully add the top.

4. Shake the bottle well to incorporate the salt and oils.

5. Wait for mixture to cool before applying to hair.

6. Shake well before use.*

how to use Spray all over hair and air-dry for light texture and some shimmer. Spray all over hair, scrunch hair in hands, and let air dry for even beachier waves.

* It is natural for the ingredients to separate. Shake well to fully combine all the ingredients before spraying.

finesse this mess detangler

Life is full of ups and downs, just like the waves in your hair. Don't let those knotty tangles mess with your mojo and ensure that your hair-brushing experience is as pain-free as possible.

what you will need

- 16-oz (480-ml) spray bottle
- Funnel
- 1¾ cups (420 ml) distilled water
- 2 tbsp (30 ml) vegetable glycerin

- 1 tbsp (15 ml) argan oil
- 1 tsp apple cider vinegar
- 20 drops jojoba oil
- 1 tsp fractionated coconut oil

MAKES ONE 16-OUNCE (480-ML) BOTTLE

step by step

1. Using the funnel, transfer the water, vegetable glycerin, argan oil, apple cider vinegar, jojoba oil, and fractionated coconut oil to the spray bottle.

2. Replace the spray top lid and shake well.*

how to use Spray liberally on clean, towel-dried hair. Use a wide-tooth comb to detangle.

* It is natural for the ingredients to separate. Shake well to fully combine all the ingredients before spraying.

sleek and clean
softening shampoo

Washing your hair shouldn't be a chore. This shampoo provides your hair with ingredients to clean away the toxins of the environment (a big thank-you to castile soap and apple cider vinegar for their hair-cleaning properties) and rejuvenates hair moisture with rose water, honey, and almond oil. Customize the scent of this shampoo to match your taste.

what you will need

- 16-oz (480-ml) bottle with pump top
- Funnel
- 1 cup (240 ml) liquid castile soap
- ½ cup (120 ml) rose water
- ½ cup (120 ml) distilled water
- 1 tsp almond oil
- 1 tsp apple cider vinegar
- 1 tsp aloe vera gel
- 1 tsp honey
- 30 drops essential oil of your choice

MAKES ONE 16-OUNCE (480-ML) BOTTLE

step by step

1. Using a funnel, put all the ingredients—adding the distilled water last—into the bottle. Fill to the top and discard any remaining water.

2. Screw on the bottle top. Shake well until all the ingredients are incorporated. *

It is natural for the ingredients to separate. Shake well to fully combine all the ingredients before using.

how to use Wet head and use one or two squirts of shampoo on hair. Start with the scalp and work your way down to the ends of your hair. Rinse well.

tip It may take a week or two for your hair to adjust to a natural shampoo. Your scalp may produce more or less oil as it adjusts. Stick with it! Your scalp should adjust to the product around week 2.

modification You can get creative with different shampoo scents. Do you like to wash your hair in the morning? Try adding citrus essential oils. Do you shower at night? Use soothing lavender or chamomile for a calming wash.

feather my tresses conditioner

Longing for an entirely new look? This ultra-nourishing conditioner will give your hair renewed volume and stylability. Nature's hydrators—including aloe, coconut oil, and vitamin E oil—will coat your hair with a soft shine. You can also customize the fragrance of your conditioner to suit your personal taste, but you might find that the intoxicating scent of rose water is enough.

what you will need

- 16-oz (480-ml) bottle with pump top
- Funnel
- ¾ cup (180 ml) rose water
- 1 tsp aloe vera gel

- 1 tsp fractionated coconut oil
- 1 tsp vegetable glycerin
- 1 tsp vitamin E oil
- 1¼ cups (300 ml) distilled water

MAKES ONE 16-OUNCE (480-ML) BOTTLE

HAIR

step by step

1. Using a funnel, put all the ingredients—adding the water last—into the bottle. Fill to the top and discard any remaining water.

2. Screw on the bottle top. Shake well until all the ingredients are incorporated.*

how to use After shampooing hair and rinsing, squeeze out excess water. Take two pumps of the conditioner and work into your hair, starting from the ends and ending with the roots. Rinse well.

tip If you want the conditioner to really take effect, leave it on for 5 minutes. For serious hydration, you can also use this as a hair mask and leave it on for 30 to 45 minutes before rinsing.

modification Did you customize your shampoo with essential oils? Use the same oils in your conditioner for a matching hair care set!

* It is natural for the ingredients to separate. Shake well to fully combine all the ingredients before using.

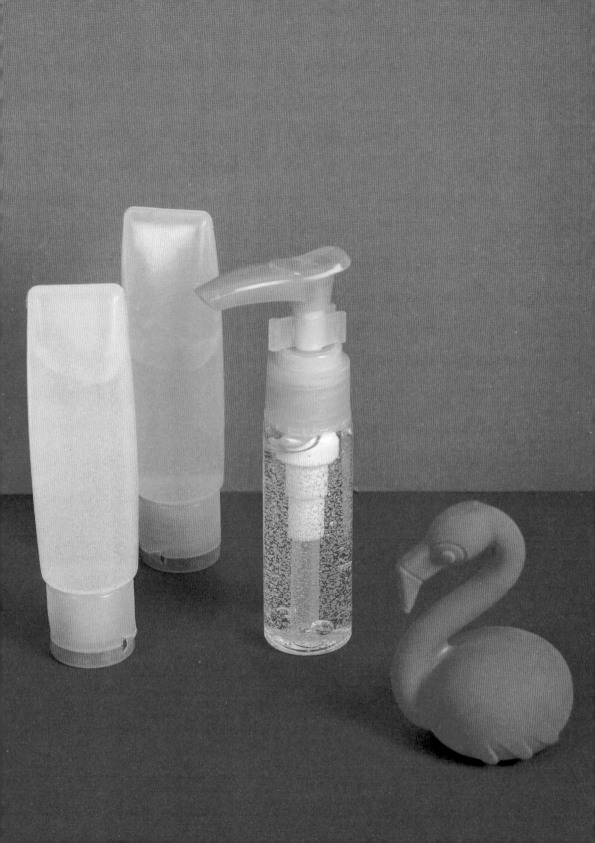

shower in a jar dry shampoo

To extend time between washings, use this dry shampoo for an effortless volumizing effect. With a little bit of this brushed on your roots, you can get that just-washed look. As an added bonus, the cinnamon helps promote healthy hair growth by stimulating the scalp.

what you will need

- 8-oz (240-ml) jar with lid
- Clean fluffy makeup brush
- 6 tbsp (48 g) arrowroot powder
- 5 tbsp (40 g) cornstarch
- 1 tsp baking soda
- ½ tsp ground cinnamon
- 10 drops grapefruit essential oil
- 10 drops ylang ylang essential oil
- 1 tbsp (15 ml) kaolin clay (for light hair)*
- 1 to 4 tbsp (8 to 32 g) Moroccan ghassoul clay (for dark hair)*

MAKES ONE 8-OUNCE (240-ML) JAR

step by step

1. Put all the ingredients in the jar.

2. Close the jar and shake until all the ingredients are fully incorporated.

how to use Lightly brush this dry shampoo onto oily areas of your hair. Focus on the areas around your hairline and in your part to keep your hair looking fresh and clean. Work into your scalp with a brush until the oils are absorbed.

* For brunettes, add more/less Moroccan ghassoul clay based on hair darkness.

shimmy shimmy coconut leave-in conditioner

This leave-in conditioner harnesses the natural power of coconut water to provide light hydration that lasts, but still gives your hair room to shimmy! Now hit the dance floor and show off your shiny locks.

what you will need

- 16-oz (480-ml) glass spray bottle
- Funnel
- 1 cup (240 ml) coconut water
- ¾ cup (180 ml) distilled water
- 20 drops vitamin E oil
- 1 tsp vegetable glycerin
- 1 tbsp (15 ml) aloe vera gel

MAKES ONE 16-OUNCE (480-ML) BOTTLE

step by step

1. Pour all the ingredients into a saucepan on the stove over low heat. Stir until the ingredients are fully incorporated. Remove from the heat.

2. Let the mixture cool to room temperature.

3. Use a funnel to transfer the mixture to the spray bottle.

how to use Use on clean damp hair. Spray all over, focusing on the ends, and brush through.

sunshine hair mask

For hair as bright and radiant as a celestial body, indulge yourself with this shine-boosting mask. All of these ingredients—avocado, honey, coconut oil, and strawberries—have natural shine-enhancing properties. They are also hydrating, so they help repair dry hair with essential fats and amino acids.

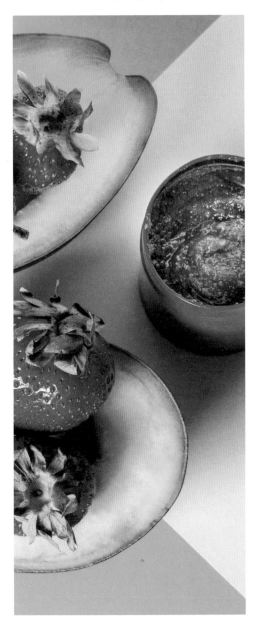

what you will need

- 8-oz (240-ml) glass jar with lid
- Double boiler*
- 1 avocado, peeled and pitted
- 1 tbsp (15 g) honey
- 5 strawberries
- 1 tbsp (15 g) coconut oil

MAKES ONE MASK

step by step

1. Mash the avocado, honey, and strawberries in a mixing bowl until fully incorporated.

2. Melt coconut oil in a double boiler over medium heat. Remove from the heat and allow to slightly cool.

3. Pour the coconut oil over the mixture and stir well until fully incorporated.

how to use Cover clean, towel-dried hair with the mask, cover with a shower cap, and leave on for 30 minutes before rinsing thoroughly out of hair.

tip The longer you leave this mask on your hair, the deeper the ingredients are able to penetrate. Put this hair mask on and watch a movie; 90 minutes later your hair will be extra glossy.

modification You can add an egg white in step 3 for extra shine.

* See page 18 for instructions.

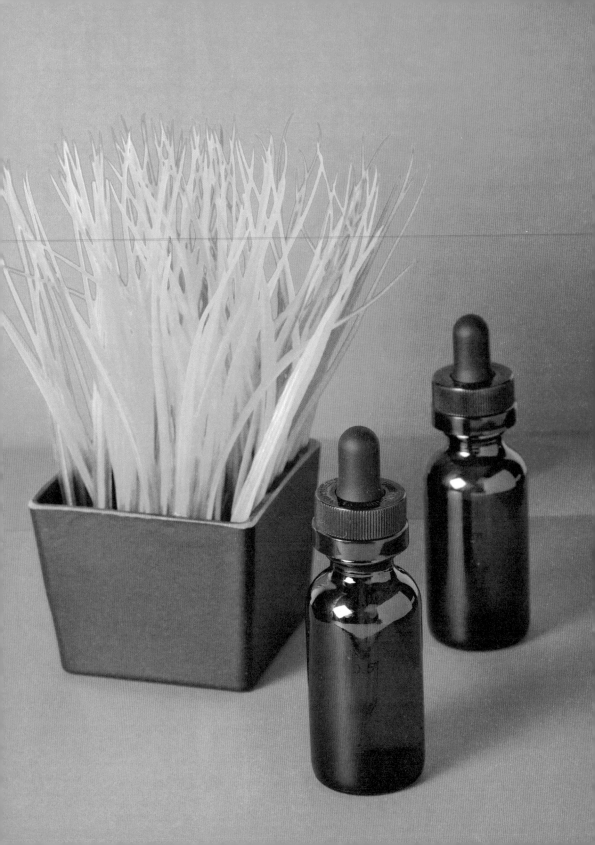

hair extraordinaire oil

A little bit of this luxurious oil goes a long way. Four super oils—argan, coconut, macadamia, and almond—collide in this hair oil that works on all hair types. A few drops will help smooth flyaways and lock in shine. A few drops more and you can pull your hair into a sleek ponytail that will stay all day without feeling sticky.

what you will need

- **4-oz (120-ml) bottle with dropper lid**
- **Funnel**
- **2 tbsp (30 ml) argan oil**

- **3 tbsp (45 ml) fractionated coconut oil**
- **2 tbsp (30 ml) macadamia oil**
- **1 tbsp (15 ml) almond oil**

MAKES ONE 4-OUNCE (120-ML) BOTTLE

step by step

1. Using a funnel, transfer all of the oils to the bottle.

2. Put on the lid and shake well until all the oils are incorporated.

how to use This can be used on wet or dry hair. Put a few drops in your palms and rub together to warm the oil. Then lightly run your hands over your hair, starting at the ends of the hair, where more moisture is needed.

tip This oil is great to use to protect your hair on a hot summer day. Going to the beach? Put a double dose of this oil on damp hair and tie in a low bun to protect it from the sun. This oil can also be used at any time on the ends of dry hair to make hair look healthy—like you got a fresh trim!

modification You can add any fragrant essential oil of your choice to this mixture for a lovely light hair perfume. Looking to give your hair an extra boost of shine? Add ⅛ tsp of mica powder (gold or iridescent for lighter hair shades, bronze for darker hair shades) to this oil and shake well before applying to hair.

new hair, new you hair mask

This quick treatment helps remove hair-dulling product buildup and coats the follicles so that hair is left shiny and smooth instead of feeling stripped. Use this mask once a month to keep hair healthy and free of buildup.

what you will need

- **2 egg whites**
- **¼ cup (60 ml) lemon juice**

MAKES ONE MASK

step by step

1. Pour the egg whites and lemon juice into a mixing bowl.

2. Whip until slightly fluffy and fully incorporated.

how to Use Apply to towel-dried clean hair. Avoid the scalp. Leave on for 10 minutes. Rinse thoroughly.

tip How does this brighten dull hair? The lemon juice breaks down shine-killing buildup while the egg white replaces the sheen.

modification You can add ½ tsp of apple cider vinegar if you're looking for an extra clarifying mask. You can also add a few drops of any essential oil of your choice to mask the slight scent of the egg whites.

no days off hair mask

If you are trying to grow out your hair—or if you already have long locks—you know that strength is key. The nourishing properties of coconut and honey meet the hair growth–boosting powers of cinnamon in this hair-strengthening trifecta.

what you will need

- **2 tbsp (30 g) coconut oil**
- **2 tbsp (30 ml) honey**
- **1 tsp ground cinnamon**

MAKES ONE MASK

step by step

1. Melt the coconut oil in a small pot on the stove over low heat. Remove from the heat.

2. Add the honey and cinnamon. Stir until fully incorporated.

how to use After shampooing, towel-dry hair. Apply the hair mask for 15 minutes. Rinse thoroughly.

tip To assist this strengthening mask, skip the hair dryer. Let your hair air-dry for a much-needed break from heat damage.

modification Add a small banana to this mask for additional strengthening benefits.

HAIR

detox your locks scalp cleanser

Even with proper shampooing and conditioning of the hair, the scalp can collect buildup in the form of leftover hair product or skin (hello, dandruff!). To beat the buildup, use this scalp detox every 2 weeks until your scalp feels free of debris. Your hair will thank you.

what you will need

- 1 tsp apple cider vinegar
- 2 tbsp (16 g) baking soda
- 1 tsp lemon juice
- 10 drops vitamin E oil
- ¼ cup (60 ml) distilled water
- 10 drops tea tree oil

MAKES ONE SCALP TREATMENT

step by step

1. Combine all the ingredients in a mixing bowl. Stir until it forms a paste.

how to use Massage the mixture into your scalp. Leave on for 30 minutes before shampooing.

tip If you have a bathtub, you can put this on your scalp before you soak. The hot water and steam from the tub will help your scalp better absorb the cleanser. Really looking to get your scalp squeaky clean? Use a silicone brush to massage the treatment deeply into the scalp for an ultra-exfoliating effect.

modification If you have a lot of product buildup, add an extra ¼ tsp of apple cider vinegar. If you have a dry scalp that is prone to dandruff, double the amount of vitamin E oil and tea tree oil. Is dandruff a big problem? Add 10 drops of bacteria-busting lavender oil to help battle flakes.

domino effect hair mask

This is the perfect mask to use when all your hair wants to do is play games. Allow yourself to relax while this sweet-smelling treatment soaks into your hair and hydrates it deeply. The longer you allow this mask to stay on your hair, the more effective it will be.

what you will need

- 1 tbsp (12 g) raw cane sugar
- 1 tbsp (15 ml) olive oil
- 1 tbsp (15 ml) coconut milk
- 1 banana
- ⅓ cup (80 g) plain yogurt
- 2 tbsp (30 ml) honey

MAKES ONE ONE MASK

step by step

1. Pour all the ingredients into a mixing bowl.
2. Mash until fully incorporated.

how to use Rub all over clean, dry hair. Twist your hair up into a bun and cover your head with a shower cap. Leave the treatment on for 45 minutes. Rinse well in the shower.

tip You can heat this mixture slightly in the microwave and apply it to your hair while warm for a deeply penetrating hydration treatment. This mixture can also be applied to warm, damp hair. Immediately apply mixture and wrap head snugly in plastic wrap to help the mixture work its magic.

modification For hydration with a shot of shine, add 10 drops of argan oil to this mask. For even more moisture-locking power that still smells good enough to eat, add ⅛ tsp of macadamia nut oil to the mixture for locks that shine.

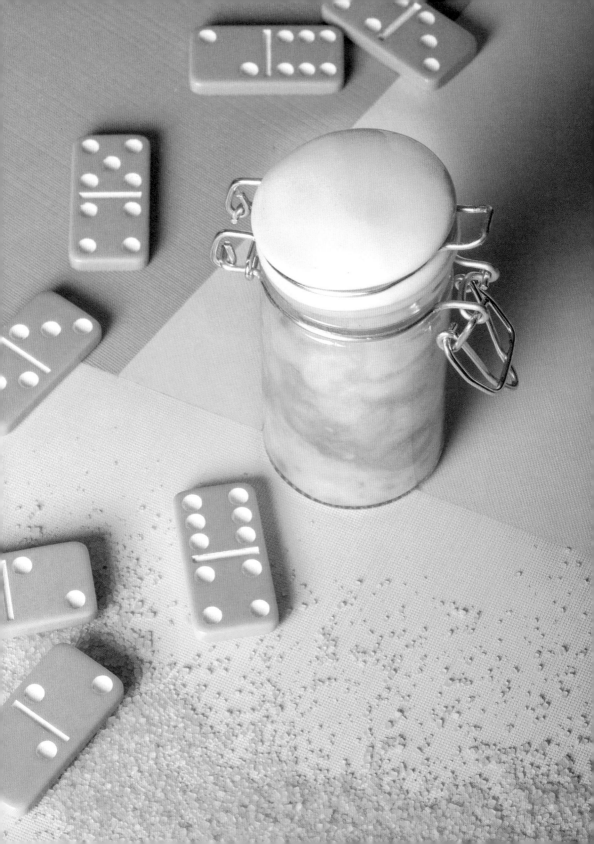

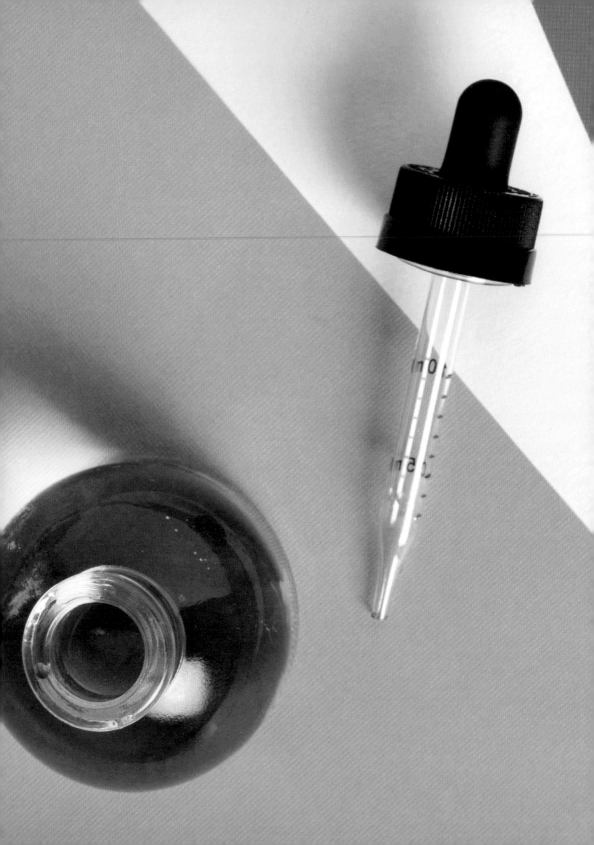

BODY

No need to Photoshop or Facetune!
Having a solid list of products that you
can count on for your body is essential.
That's why we've created these recipes
that will hopefully boost your confidence
and your health. With items like
sunscreen, shower products, perfumes,
and oils, we're here for you. So what are
you waiting for? It's time for a glow-up!

coffee break body scrub

Instead of having your morning caffeine in a cup, have it in the shower! This coffee-based scrub uses caffeine to energize, plump, and smooth your skin. The natural exfoliating abilities of the brown sugar and sea salt remove rough skin for a baby-soft finish. The macadamia oil and almond oil pack a hydrating one-two punch to get your day started right.

what you will need

- 8-oz (240-ml) jar with lid
- 3 tbsp (45 g) sea salt
- 4 tbsp (50 g) raw cane sugar
- 5 tbsp (40 g) coffee grounds
- 2 tbsp (30 ml) almond oil
- 1 tbsp (15 ml) macadamia oil

MAKES ONE 8-OUNCE (240-ML) JAR

step by step

1. Put the salt, sugar, and coffee grounds in the jar.

2. Put the lid on the jar and shake to combine the ingredients.

3. Take off the lid and add the almond oil and macadamia oil.

4. Put the lid back on the jar and shake well to incorporate the oil with the dry ingredients.

how to use You can use this as a dry scrub for deep exfoliation or as a wet scrub for gentle exfoliation and hydration. For a dry scrub, step into the shower and rub the mixture in a circular motion all over your body. Rinse off with warm water. For a wet scrub, after washing your body in the shower, rub the scrub all over your wet body. Rinse off with warm water.

tip Looking for extra hydration after you exfoliate? Keep the scrub on your skin for at least 5 minutes before rinsing it off. This gives the almond oil and macadamia oil time to really sink in and gives the coffee some time to provide your skin with an extra caffeine pick-me-up!

modification For an extra morning boost, add some orange oil for a shock of citrus or eucalyptus oil for a tingly exfoliating experience.

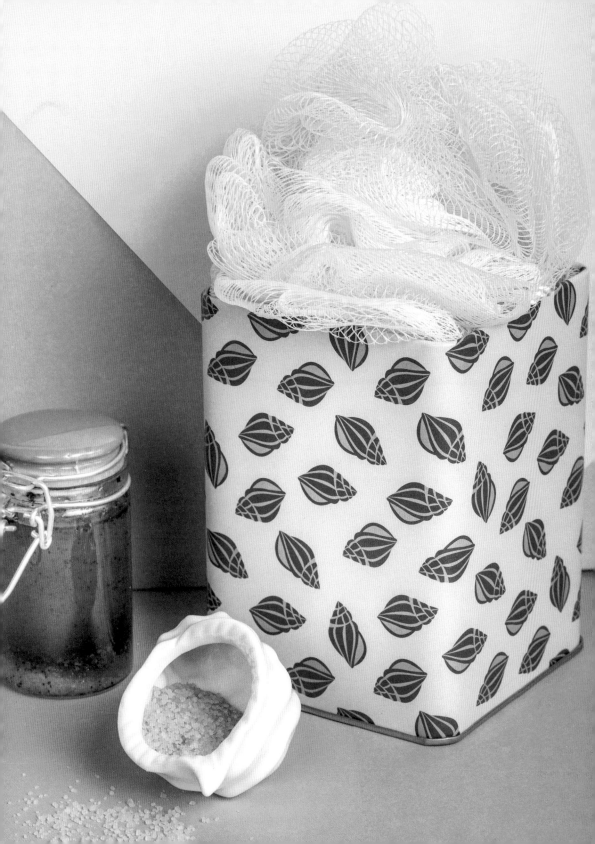

you glow, girl sunscreen

The sun can pose some serious dangers if you don't protect your skin. This sunscreen is a major multitasker—it provides natural sun protection while heavily hydrating and nourishing the skin with coconut oil, aloe vera gel, and shea butter. And because every goddess deserves to shine, this sunscreen adds just a touch of a bronze glow with natural mica powder.

what you will need

- 8-oz (240-ml) glass jar with lid
- Double boiler*
- 6 tbsp (90 g) coconut oil
- 2 tbsp (30 g) shea butter
- 3 tbsp (45 g) white beeswax pellets
- 2 tsp aloe vera gel (clear)

- 1 tbsp (15 g) zinc oxide
- 1 tsp almond oil
- 2 tsp red raspberry oil
- 1 tsp carrot seed oil
- ½ tsp mica powder (bronze)

MAKES ONE 8-OUNCE (240-ML) JAR

BODY

step by step

1. Heat the coconut oil, shea butter, and white beeswax pellets in a double boiler over medium heat until all the ingredients are completely melted.

2. Once melted, remove from the heat, add the aloe vera gel, and stir until incorporated.

3. Allow the mixture to cool slightly.

4. While the mixture is still warm, add the zinc oxide, almond oil, red raspberry oil, carrot seed oil, and mica powder. Stir well.

5. Pour the warm mixture into the jar and carefully add the lid. Put in the freezer for 30 minutes to harden.

how to use Apply all over your face and body before sun exposure. This formula isn't waterproof, so reapply frequently throughout the day if you take a dip in the water or perspire in the sun.

tip Don't forget sensitive spots like the exposed parts of your scalp, your ears, and the tops of your feet!

sun safety Zinc oxide provides a heavy dose of natural SPF, but so does the coconut oil, red raspberry seed oil, and carrot seed oil!

modification This works beautifully as a daily lotion. Just double the amount of shea butter for a shimmery lotion with built-in sun protection.

See page 18 for instructions.

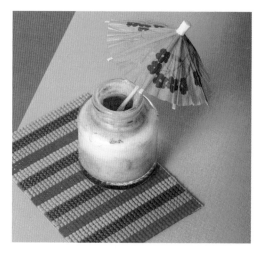

beach, please! sunscreen

This product can double as a moisturizer, so lather up and share it with your whole beach party. Increase the amount of zinc oxide to boost the ray-fighting abilities of this super sunscreen.

what you will need

- 8-oz (240-ml) glass jar with lid
- Double boiler*
- 6 tbsp (90 g) coconut oil
- 2 tbsp (30 g) shea butter
- 3 tbsp (45 g) white beeswax pellets
- 1 tbsp (15 g) zinc oxide
- 1 tsp kukui oil
- 20 drops ylang ylang oil

MAKES ONE 8-OUNCE (240-ML) JAR

step by step

1. Heat the coconut oil, shea butter, and white beeswax pellets in a double boiler over medium heat until all the ingredients are completely melted.

2. Once melted, remove from the heat and allow the mixture to cool slightly.

3. While the mixture is still warm, add the zinc oxide, kukui oil, and ylang ylang oil. Stir well.

4. Pour the warm mixture into the jar and carefully add the lid. Put in the freezer to harden.

how to use Apply to face and body before sun exposure. Reapply as needed.

tip The ylang ylang oil in the sunscreen is a fragrance that is subtle enough for the beach, but also sophisticated enough for brunch. Use this ultra-hydrating sunscreen daily as a sun protector that doubles as an everyday moisturizer.

See page 18 for instructions.

BODY

destination relaxation soak

Having trouble relaxing at the end of the day? Try this calming soak to help signal to your mind and body that bedtime is around the corner. You'll be ready to drift off to dreamland in no time.

what you will need

- 8-oz (240-ml) jar with lid
- ¼ cup (60 g) Epsom salt
- ¼ cup (60 g) sea salt
- 30 drops lavender oil
- 20 drops chamomile oil

MAKES ONE 8-OUNCE (240-ML) JAR

step by step

1. Put the Epsom salt and sea salt in the jar. Screw on the lid and shake well.

2. Remove the lid. Add the lavender oil and chamomile oil to the salt. Screw on the lid and shake well.

how to use Add two heaping scoops to warm bathwater and stir until dissolved. Soak for 20 minutes before rinsing your body.

tip Try to take this soak an hour before bedtime to give your mind time to unplug and your body time to unwind.

modification You can also add 10 drops of bergamot oil for even more stress-busting strength.

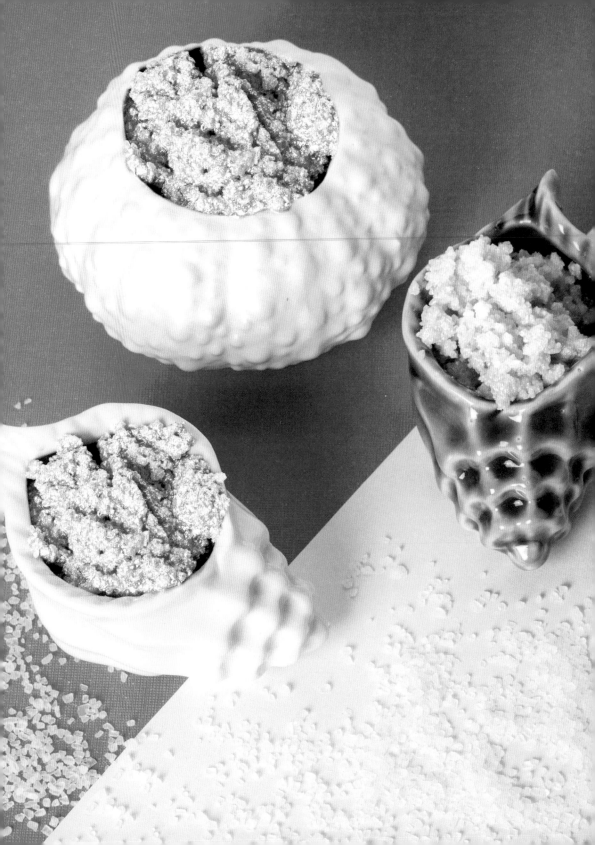

under the sea scrub

This iridescent coconut-based scrub will transport you to a magical world under the sea. Sweet coconut sugar and pearlescent mica powder will make you feel as if you have emerged from a mermaid's paradise: you will smell sweet, your body will be baby-smooth, and you will shine when the sun hits your skin.

what you will need

- 8-oz (240-ml) jar with lid
- 5 tbsp (75 g) finely ground sea salt
- 7 tbsp (95 g) coconut palm sugar

- 1 tsp mica powder (iridescent)
- 2 tbsp (30 ml) fractionated coconut oil

MAKES ONE 8-OUNCE (240-ML) JAR

step by step

1. Put the salt, sugar, and mica powder in the jar.

2. Put the lid on the jar and shake to combine the ingredients.

3. Take off the lid and add the fractionated coconut oil.

4. Put the lid back on the jar and shake well to incorporate the oil with the dry ingredients.

how to use After washing your body in the shower, rub the scrub all over your wet skin. Rinse off with warm water.

tip If you want the shimmer to stick to your skin after your shower, use this exfoliator as the last step of your showering routine. Rinse off and pat your body dry.

modification Want to make the experience even more magical? Add more mica powder to the scrub. You can leave your shower feeling like a dewy disco ball.

super citrus scrub

This is the perfect scrub to get your day started. The lemon and grapefruit oils signal to your brain that it's time to spring into action. The salt, sugar, and coconut oil provide exfoliation and hydration simultaneously, saving you precious morning minutes. Now go change the world!

what you will need

- 8-oz (240-ml) jar with lid
- 5 tbsp (75 g) finely ground sea salt
- 7 tbsp (95 g) raw cane sugar
- 2 tbsp (30 ml) fractionated coconut oil
- 20 drops lemon oil
- 20 drops grapefruit oil

MAKES ONE 8-OUNCE (240-ML) JAR

step by step

1. Put the salt and sugar in the jar.

2. Put the lid on the jar and shake to combine the ingredients.

3. Take off the lid and add the fractionated coconut oil, lemon oil, and grapefruit oil.

4. Put the lid back on the jar and shake well to incorporate the oil with the dry ingredients.

how to use Rub all over your body for an invigorating scrub that smooths and softens. Rub the scrub into dry skin before your shower for a deeper exfoliating experience. Apply the scrub to damp skin from the shower for a gentler exfoliation.

tip Dry-rub first thing in the morning with this wake-you-up scrub. The citrus essential oils help start the day off with a burst of energy.

modification If you're looking to use this scrub at night, use lavender and bergamot instead of citrus oils. If you'd like to use this scrub as a soak, replace the cane sugar with Epsom salt.

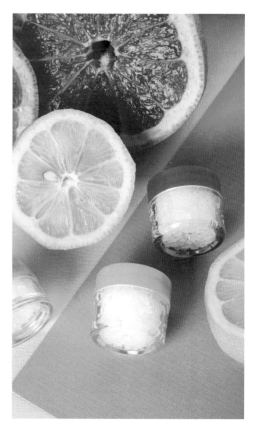

walk a mile in your louboutins foot soak

Let your feet relax in this healing and hydrating super-soak. Epsom salts help soothe achy arches, and shea butter, honey, and jojoba oil work together to soften rough skin. Follow this soak with a foot lotion to lock in the deep hydration.

what you will need

- 8-oz (240-ml) glass jar with lid
- Double boiler*
- 10 tbsp (150 g) Epsom salt
- 1 tbsp (15 ml) shea butter
- 1 tbsp (15 ml) honey
- 20 drops jojoba oil

MAKES ONE 8-OUNCE (240-ML) JAR

step by step

1. Put the Epsom salt in the jar.

2. In a double boiler over medium heat, melt the shea butter completely. Remove from the heat.

3. While the melted shea butter is still warm, add the honey. Stir until completely incorporated.

4. Add the jojoba oil to the shea butter and honey mixture. Stir until completely incorporated.

5. Pour the liquid over the Epsom salt.

6. Carefully put the lid on the jar and shake well until all the ingredients are fully incorporated.

how to use Put a heaping scoop of the mixture into a warm footbath. Stir until the mixture dissolves. Soak your feet for 20 minutes.

tip Follow this soak with a super-emulsifying lotion to lock in its hydrating effects.

modification Feet feeling tired? Add 10 drops of tea tree oil and 10 drops of peppermint oil to the soak. These essential oils help revive tired toes.

* See page 18 for instructions.

happy day bath soak

We all have those days when we feel a little "blah." Bathe your blues away in this mood-brightening soak that softens the skin and smells like a citrus grove and rose garden at the same time. Take some time to reflect, relax, and rejuvenate before moving on. After all, self-care is the new trend!

what you will need

- 8-oz (240-ml) jar with lid
- ¼ cup (60 g) Epsom salt
- ¼ cup (60 g) sea salt
- 10 drops lemon oil
- 30 drops grapefruit oil
- 10 drops rose oil

MAKES ONE 8-OUNCE (240-ML) JAR

step by step

1. Put the Epsom salt and sea salt in the jar. Screw on the lid and shake well.

2. Remove the lid. Add the lemon oil, grapefruit oil, and rose oil to the salt. Screw on the lid and shake well.

how to use Add two heaping scoops to warm bathwater and stir until dissolved. Soak for 20 minutes before rinsing your body.

tip Turn this mood-brightening moment into an opportunity for self-care. Pair this soak with a face mask and hair mask for a major mood lift. This coarse mixture can also double as a soak and a dry-body scrub. Stand in a bathtub full of warm water and, instead of dumping the soak directly into the bath water, grab two handfuls and rub it over your dry body for an immediate exfoliating effect. Then sit down to soak and allow any remaining mixture to dissolve in the water.

modification If you're looking to use this scrub at night, switch out the citrus oils for lavender and bergamot. If you'd like to use this scrub as a soak, replace the Epsom salt with raw cane sugar. Looking for something a little more floral? Switch out the rose oil with jasmine oil for an intoxicating scent.

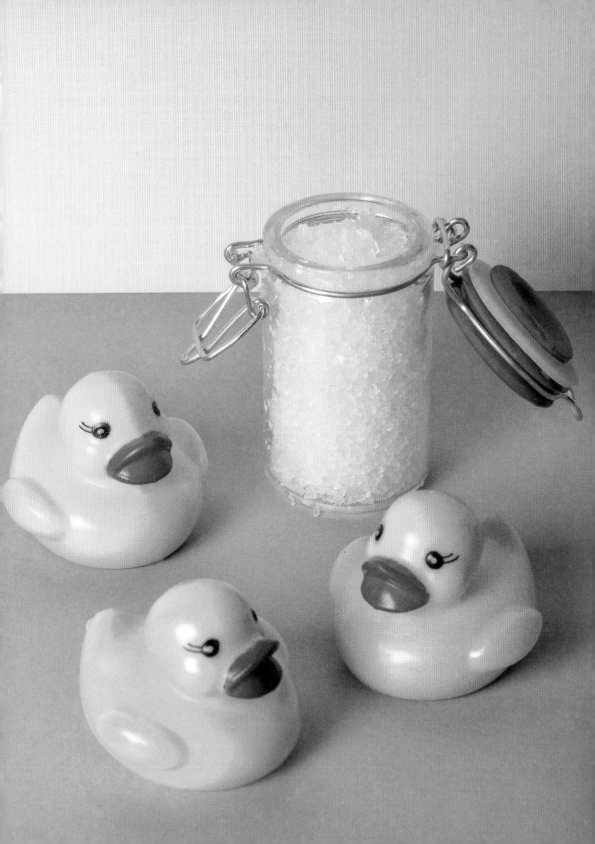

cosmic calm bodywash

Get yourself ready for dreamtime with this relaxing bodywash. It harnesses the pacifying properties of lavender and bergamot and wraps them up with soothing rose water. You'll be getting a visit from Mr. Sandman as soon as your head hits the pillow.

what you will need

- 16-oz (480-ml) bottle with pump top
- Funnel
- 3 tbsp (45 ml) aloe vera gel
- ½ cup (120 ml) rose water
- ½ cup (120 ml) distilled water
- ¾ cup (180 ml) liquid castile soap
- 3 tsp vitamin E oil
- 40 drops lavender oil
- 20 drops bergamot oil

MAKES ONE 16-OUNCE (480-ML) BOTTLE

step by step

1. Using a funnel, put all the ingredients into the bottle.

2. Screw on the bottle top. Shake well until all the ingredients are incorporated.

how to use Apply two pumps to a wet loofah and work into a lather. Scrub all over your body. Avoid the face and eyes. Rinse your body thoroughly.

tip Before scrubbing, deeply inhale the scent of the bodywash on the loofah five times. This will help you reap the benefits of the lavender and bergamot and signal to your body that it's time to wind down for the night.

modification You can switch out the bergamot oil for chamomile oil for another soothing bedtime blend.

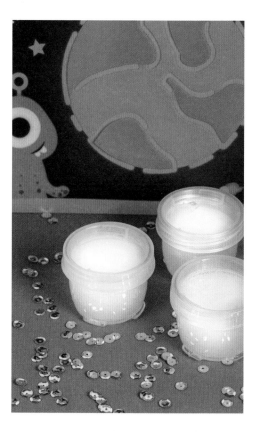

get up and glow bodywash

This rose- and citrus-scented bodywash will motivate and invigorate. The aromatherapy benefits of grapefruit and lemon will help improve your mood.

what you will need

- 16-oz (480-ml) bottle with pump top
- Funnel
- 3 tbsp (45 ml) aloe vera gel
- ½ cup (120 ml) rose water
- ½ cup (120 ml) distilled water
- ¾ cup (180 ml) liquid castile soap
- 3 tsp vitamin E oil
- 30 drops grapefruit oil
- 30 drops lemon oil

MAKES ONE 16-OUNCE (480-ML) BOTTLE

step by step

1. Using a funnel, put all the ingredients into the bottle.

2. Screw on the bottle top. Shake well until all the ingredients are incorporated.

how to use Apply two pumps to a wet loofah and work into a lather. Scrub all over your body. Avoid the face and eyes. Rinse your body thoroughly.

tip If you like to take a bath instead of a shower, you can use this bodywash as a sweet-smelling bubble bath.

BODY

sweat-be-gone salve

The baking soda in this recipe stops the odors before they start.

what you will need

- 8-oz (240-ml) glass jar with lid
- Double boiler*
- 5 tbsp (75 ml) coconut oil
- 4 tbsp (60 g) shea butter
- 2 tbsp (16 g) arrowroot powder
- 1 tbsp (8 g) baking soda
- 1 tbsp (8 g) kaolin clay

MAKES ONE 8-OUNCE (240-ML) JAR

See page 18 for instructions.

step by step

1. In a double boiler over medium heat, melt the coconut oil and shea butter. Remove from the heat.

2. While the mixture is warm, add the arrowroot powder, baking soda, and kaolin clay. Stir well.

3. Pour the warm mixture into the jar and carefully add the lid.

4. Put in the freezer for 30 minutes to harden.

how to use Rub a layer onto dry underarms. Reapply as needed.

garden party deodorant

This super hydrating floral deodorant doubles as a light perfume. Vitamin E oil keeps extra-sensitive skin moisturized while still protecting against any unwelcome aromas. Bonus: You can apply it right after shaving your underarms, as the vitamin E oil will stop further irritation.

what you will need

- 8-oz (240-ml) glass jar with lid
- Double boiler*
- Funnel
- 5 tbsp (75 ml) coconut oil
- 4 tbsp (60 g) shea butter
- 1 tbsp (8 g) arrowroot powder

- 1 tbsp (8 g) baking soda
- 1 tbsp (8 g) kaolin clay
- 10 drops rose oil
- 20 drops jasmine oil
- ½ tsp vitamin E oil

MAKES ONE 8-OUNCE (240-ML) JAR

step by step

1. In a double boiler over medium heat, melt the coconut oil and shea butter. Remove from the heat.

2. While the mixture is warm, add the arrowroot powder, baking soda, kaolin clay, rose oil, jasmine oil, and vitamin E oil. Stir well.

3. Pour the warm mixture into the jar and carefully add the lid.

4. Put immediately into the freezer for 30 minutes to harden.

how to use Apply to clean and dry underarms.

tip The scent of jasmine oils can vary greatly depending on the manufacturer. Try a variety of jasmine oils until you find the one you love.

modification Don't be afraid to try mixing your own floral blend.

* See page 18 for instructions.

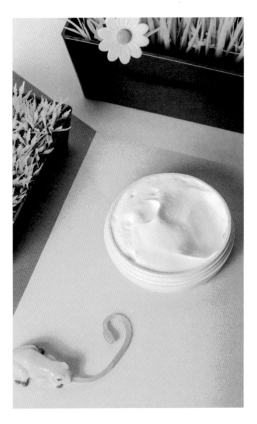

silky smooth body lotion

This hydrating lotion harnesses the magical properties of vegetable glycerin, which naturally binds water to the skin. The light and bright scent of grapefruit oil and the slight sheen of coconut oil make this the perfect everyday lotion.

what you will need

- 8-oz (240-ml) glass jar with lid
- Double boiler*
- 6 tbsp (90 ml) coconut oil
- 4 tbsp (60 g) shea butter

- 1 tbsp (15 ml) vegetable glycerin
- 1 tbsp (15 ml) almond oil
- 30 drops grapefruit oil

MAKES ONE 8-OUNCE (240-ML) JAR

step by step

1. In a double boiler over medium heat, melt the coconut oil and shea butter. Remove from the heat.

2. While the mixture is warm, add the vegetable glycerin, almond oil, and grapefruit oil. Stir well.

3. Pour the warm mixture into the jar and carefully add the lid.

4. Put immediately in the freezer for 30 minutes to harden.

how to use Apply all over your body.

tip Apply while just dry from the shower to lock in extra moisture. This lotion can also be applied to hair if you want a sleek look. Take 1 tsp of the lotion and run it through your hair before placing it in a low ponytail or bun.

modification The citrusy scent of the grapefruit isn't your thing? Try rosemary for an unexpected and elegantly earthy note or sandalwood for a gender-neutral aroma. If you'd like to give your body lotion a little extra shine, double the amount of almond oil for a glowy sheen.

* See page 18 for instructions.

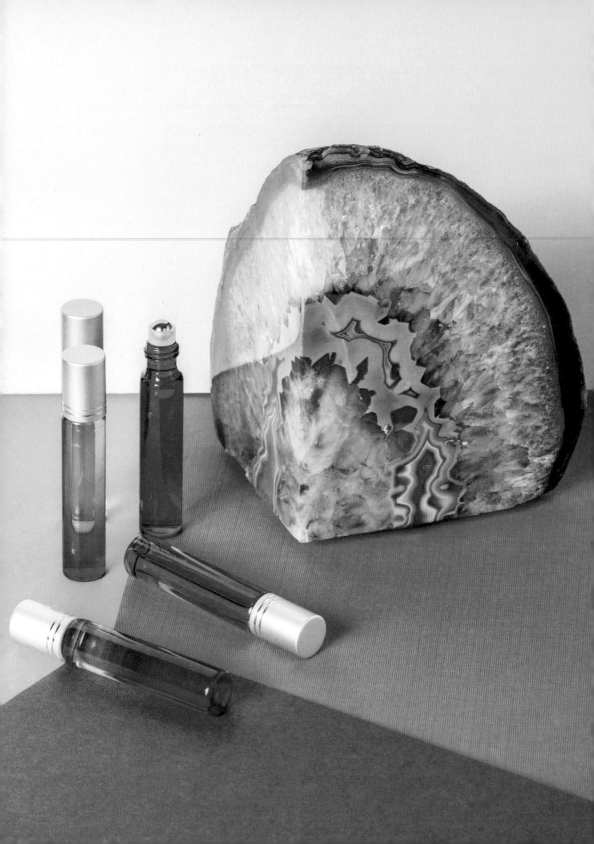

rare earth fragrance

The unexpected inclusion of basil oil in a floral perfume balances the syrupy sweetness of intoxicating jasmine and gardenia oils with an earthy element. This twist on a classic floral perfume is a great signature scent.

what you will need

- 15 ml roll-on bottle
- Funnel
- 100 drops jojoba oil

- 75 drops jasmine oil
- 50 drops gardenia oil
- 25 drops basil oil

MAKES ONE 15 ML BOTTLE

step by step

1. Using the funnel, put the jojoba oil in the bottle.

2. Place the jasmine oil, gardenia oil, and basil oil in the bottle.

3. Screw on the roll-on top and the cap. Shake well.

how to use Apply to clean, dry skin.

tip A little goes a long way. If you are wearing your hair up, put this perfume on the nape of your neck. You'll leave a trail of sweet-smelling earthy magic wherever you go. Want the scent to be super subtle? Apply only behind the knees.

modification If jasmine and gardenia aren't your favorite florals, try any floral oil of your choice in lieu of the oils suggested in this recipe. If you would like a tropical twist on this scent, swap the gardenia oil for grapefruit oil.

here for hydration cream

This luxurious cream shows your hands some much-needed love.

what you will need

- 8-oz (240-ml) glass jar with lid
- Double boiler*
- 6 tbsp (90 ml) coconut oil
- 2 tbsp (30 g) shea butter
- 2 tbsp (30 g) mango butter
- 1 tsp vitamin E oil
- ½ tsp jojoba oil
- 20 drops rosemary oil

MAKES ONE 8-OUNCE (240-ML) JAR

* See page 18 for instructions.

step by step

1. In a double boiler over medium heat, melt the coconut oil, shea butter, and mango butter. Remove from the heat.

2. While the mixture is warm, add the vitamin E oil, jojoba oil, and rosemary oil. Stir well.

3. Pour the warm mixture into the jar. Wait to cool before putting on the lid.

4. Put immediately in the freezer for 30 minutes to harden.

how to use Apply to hands and forearms. Pay extra attention rubbing the lotion into the cuticles for deep hydration.

yas queen body oil

This luxurious body oil provides a natural glow with a slight floral scent.

what you will need

- 4-oz (120-ml) bottle with dropper top
- Funnel
- 2 tsp (10 ml) rosehip seed oil
- 2 tsp (10 ml) jojoba oil
- 3 tbsp (45 ml) olive oil
- 3 tbsp (45 ml) avocado oil
- 20 drops rose oil
- 2 tsp (10 ml) pomegranate oil

MAKES ONE 4-OUNCE (120-ML) BOTTLE

how to use Apply to skin while still damp from shower.

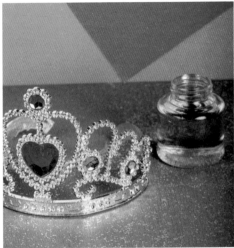

step by step

1. Use a funnel to put all the ingredients into the bottle.

2. Shake well.

pinkies up overnight
hand cream treatment

Give your hands an instant reset with this overnight treatment. Soothe tired and dry hands and knuckles with this moisture-locking, deeply penetrating lotion. Keep this treatment on your nightstand to hydrate hands before bedtime. Before you know it, your hands will be ready to wow at your next high tea!

what you will need

- 50-gram glass cosmetic container with lid
- Double boiler*
- 1 tsp shea butter
- 1 tsp white beeswax pellets
- 1½ tbsp (23 ml) coconut oil

- 1 tbsp (15 ml) vegetable glycerin
- 1 tsp jojoba oil
- 1 tsp avocado oil
- 1 tsp grapeseed oil

ONE 50-GRAM COSMETIC CONTAINER

BODY

step by step

1. In a double boiler over medium heat, melt the shea butter, white beeswax pellets, and coconut oil completely. Remove from the heat.

2. While the mixture is still warm, add the vegetable glycerin. Stir until completely incorporated.

3. Add the jojoba oil, avocado oil, and grapeseed oil. Stir until completely incorporated.

4. Transfer the mixture to the cosmetic container and carefully add the lid.

5. Immediately put the mixture in the freezer for 30 minutes to harden.

See page 18 for instructions.

how to use Apply liberally to clean, dry hands before bed.

tip For an extra hydrating overnight treatment, put on moisturizing gloves after applying the cream to your hands. The trapped heat will help it absorb even further.

another tip Looking for photo-worthy hands? First apply a cuticle treatment to clean, dry cuticles. Then apply this lotion to your hands. Then cover with moisturizing gloves. You'll wake up with super hydrated and smooth hands.

modification To make this treatment ultra-soothing before you hit the hay, add a few drops of chamomile oil for a natural way to lull yourself to sleep.

unicorn in a jar lotion

Whether you want to wear this on special occasions or feel like a fabulous mythical beast every day, this is a great lotion to add to your vanity. It's like having your own personal unicorn. This lotion can be used all over your body for hydration and glowiness from head to toe.

what you will need

- 8-oz (240-ml) glass jar with lid
- Double boiler*
- 6 tbsp (90 ml) coconut oil
- 4 tbsp (60 g) shea butter

- 1 tbsp (15 ml) aloe vera gel
- 20 drops jasmine oil
- ½ tsp mica powder (bronze)
- ¼ tsp mica powder (iridescent)

MAKES ONE 8-OUNCE (240-ML) JAR

step by step

1. In a double boiler over medium heat, melt the coconut oil and shea butter. Remove from the heat.

2. While the mixture is warm, add the aloe vera gel, jasmine oil, and mica powders. Stir well.

3. Pour the warm mixture into the jar and carefully add the lid.

4. Put immediately in the freezer for 30 minutes to harden.

how to use Use all over the body.

tip Use this lotion on legs, arms, and collarbone to add a little shine to your look. This lotion is safe to use on the face. Try using it instead of foundation for a supernatural, mega-glowing, skin-loving look.

modification You can add different colored mica powders to really make this lotion come to life. Try hot pink, teal, and green mica powder for the days when you're feeling a little wild. Mix pearlescent, silver, and gold mica powders for an ethereal glow. Is it summertime? Triple the amount of bronze mica powder for a shimmery lotion that also gives a golden glow.

See page 18 for instructions.

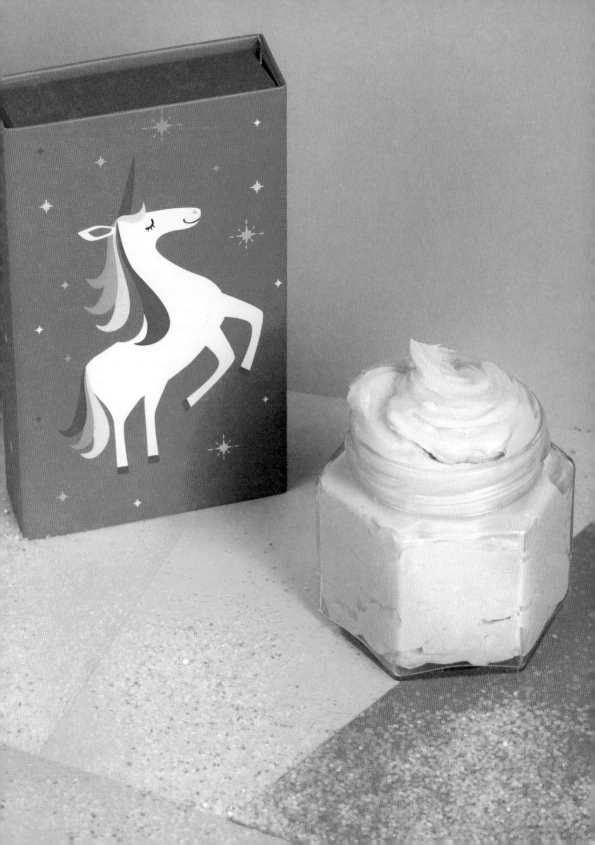

barefoot in bora bora lotion

To keep your feet sandal ready all year long, store a jar of this super-rich lotion by your bed and apply first thing in the morning. The tea tree oil provides a soothing homeopathic remedy for tired toes. The shea butter, olive oil, rosehip oil, and vegetable glycerin are mega-hydrators. This lotion also doubles as an overnight foot treatment.

what you will need

- 8-oz (240-ml) glass jar with lid
- Double boiler*
- 6 tbsp (90 ml) coconut oil
- 2 tbsp (30 g) shea butter

- 1 tbsp (15 ml) olive oil
- 1 tsp rosehip oil
- ½ tsp tea tree oil
- 1 tbsp (15 ml) vegetable glycerin

MAKES ONE 8-OUNCE (240-ML) JAR

step by step

1. In a double boiler over medium heat, melt the coconut oil and shea butter. Remove from the heat.

2. While the mixture is still warm, add the olive oil, rosehip oil, tea tree oil, and vegetable glycerin. Stir well.

3. Pour the warm mixture into the jar and carefully add the lid.

4. Put immediately in the freezer for 30 minutes to harden.

how to use Apply to feet and ankles as needed. Pay special attention to the heel area.

tip Apply a thick layer of this cream to your feet and cover with socks before bed. As the feet heat up during sleep, the lotion will absorb more deeply into the skin for an indulgent overnight treatment.

modification If you'd like an invigorating lotion, add some drops of peppermint oil to the cream for a tingly refresher for tired feet.

*See page 18 for instructions.

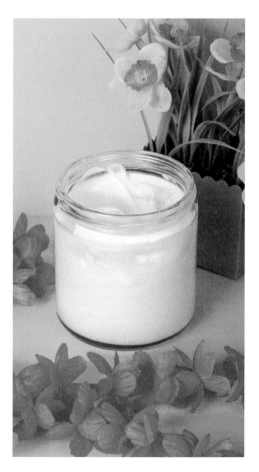

tired tootsie foot treatment

This overnight foot treatment will have you waking up thinking that you visited a foot spa in your dreams. The peppermint oil is refreshingly tingly while the shea butter, vitamin E oil, and avocado oil hydrate cracked heels and lock in moisture.

what you will need

- 8-oz (240-ml) glass jar with lid
- Double boiler*
- 2 tbsp (30 g) shea butter
- 2 tbsp (30 g) beeswax pellets
- 4 tbsp (60 ml) coconut oil
- 2 tbsp (30 ml) avocado oil
- 2 tsp vitamin E oil
- 30 drops peppermint oil

MAKES ONE 8-OUNCE (240-ML) JAR

step by step

1. In a double boiler over medium heat, melt the shea butter, beeswax pellets, and coconut oil completely. Remove from the heat.

2. While the mixture is still warm, add the avocado oil, vitamin E oil, and peppermint oil. Stir until completely incorporated.

3. Transfer the mixture to the jar and carefully add the lid.

4. Immediately put the mixture in the freezer for 30 minutes to harden.

how to use Apply liberally to clean, dry feet before bed.

tip For an extra hydrating overnight treatment, put on socks after applying the treatment to your feet. The heat will help it absorb even further. This lotion is also the perfect way to show yourself a little self-care as a foot massage.

modification This treatment doesn't need to be reserved for the evening. If you need sandal-ready feet in a flash, massage this treatment into your tootsies for 5 minutes. Immediately sandal-worthy. You can also add 10 drops of tea tree oil for added antibacterial benefits and an extra tingly sensation.

* See page 18 for instructions.

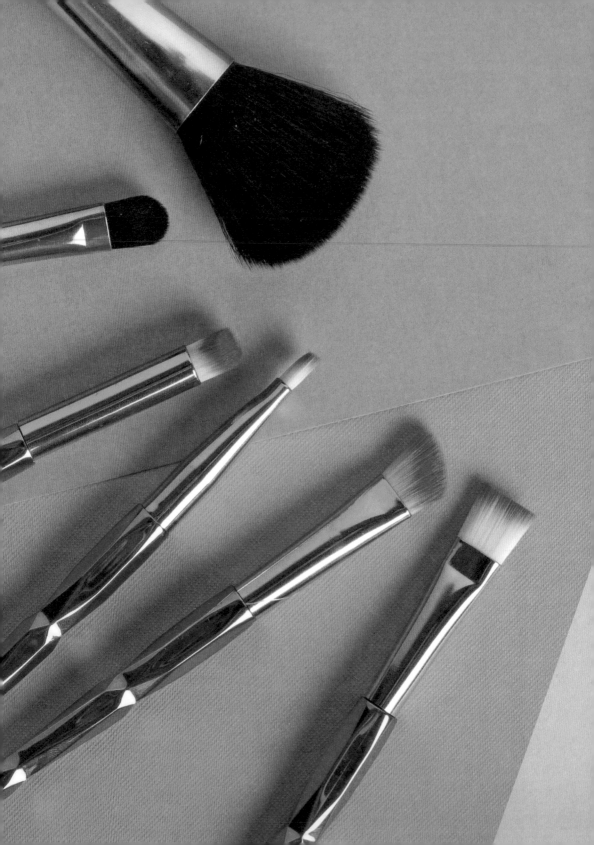

MAKEUP

Ah, makeup! The go-to of glowing goddesses and gods who want to feel glamorous on every occasion. No matter your skin tone, gender, or personality, this section has a little something for everyone. From peachy cheeks perfect for a picnic, to deep crimson lips fit to enchant, to a dewy, barely there glow, look here for recipes to help you achieve your ultimate beauty goals! The best part is, you're the one who gets to decide where you draw the line.

baby lips lip balm

Nothing ruins a vibe like dry, chapped lips. Keep your pout smooth with this nourishing balm that smells as good as it looks. Put this on the moment after you brush your teeth in the morning for lips that stay hydrated and look youthful all day long.

what you will need

- 50-gram glass cosmetic container with lid
- Double boiler*
- 1 tsp white beeswax pellets
- 2 tsp shea butter
- 2 tbsp (30 ml) coconut oil

- ¼ tsp jojoba oil
- ¼ tsp rosehip oil
- ¼ tsp vanilla extract
- 10 drops rose oil

MAKES ONE 50-GRAM CONTAINER

step by step

1. In a double boiler over medium heat, melt the white beeswax pellets, shea butter, and coconut oil. Remove from the heat.

2. While the mixture is warm, add the jojoba oil, rosehip oil, vanilla extract, and rose oil. Stir well.

3. Pour the warm mixture into the cosmetic container and carefully add the lid.

4. Put immediately in the freezer for 30 minutes to harden.

how to use Smooth onto clean and dry lips. Can be worn alone or under lipstick or lip gloss.

tip After using a lip scrub, immediately apply this lip balm to help lock in moisture.

modification If you would like a tinted lip balm, you can add some hibiscus flower powder for a light pink flush or some beetroot powder for a more intense pink pucker.

See page 18 for instructions.

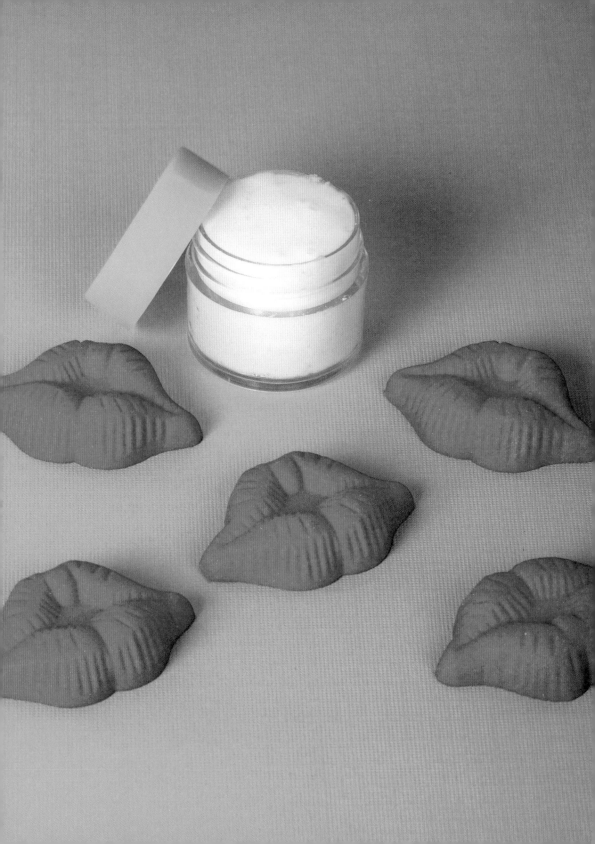

pucker-up lip mask

So many super-hydrators—mango butter, vitamin E oil, and castor oil, to name a few—come together in this powerful lip mask. You can put on this mask for 15 minutes for a quick fix, wear it all day as an ultra-emulsifying salve, or wear it overnight to wake up with the softest lips.

what you will need

- 50-gram glass cosmetic container with lid
- Double boiler*
- 2 tbsp (30 ml) coconut oil
- 1 tbsp (15 g) mango butter
- ¼ tsp castor oil
- ¼ tsp jojoba oil
- ¼ tsp vitamin E oil
- ¼ tsp sweet almond oil
- ¼ tsp macadamia nut oil

MAKES ONE 50-GRAM CONTAINER

step by step

1. In a double boiler over medium heat, melt the coconut oil and mango butter. Remove from the heat.

2. While the mixture is warm, add the castor oil, jojoba oil, vitamin E oil, sweet almond oil, and macadamia nut oil. Stir well.

3. Pour the warm mixture into the cosmetic container and carefully add the lid.

4. Put immediately in freezer for 30 minutes to harden.

how to use Apply a generous layer after brushing teeth before bed. Wear overnight.

tip Right before bed, use a lip scrub and then follow with a thick layer of this salve. It will penetrate deeply while you sleep. You will wake up to extra soft lips.

modification Super dry lips? Double the amount of vitamin E oil and castor oil for a deeply hydrating overnight treatment.

See page 18 for instructions.

milky way lip balm

This high-shine balm gets its shimmery magic from the combination of coconut oil, grapeseed oil, and the shooting star of the show: mica powder. This balm looks beautiful when worn alone, over a lip stain, or with a full face of makeup. Regardless of application, the dazzling sparkle will remind you of gazing at the cosmos.

what you will need

- 50-gram glass cosmetic container with lid
- Double boiler*
- Funnel
- 1 tsp beeswax pellets

- 2 tbsp (30 ml) coconut oil
- ¼ tsp grapeseed oil
- ½ tsp mica powder (iridescent)

MAKES ONE 50-GRAM CONTAINER

step by step

1. In a double boiler over medium heat, melt the beeswax pellets and coconut oil. Remove from the heat.

2. Add the grapeseed oil and mica powder. Stir until fully incorporated.

3. Using the funnel, transfer the mixture to the cosmetic container and carefully add the lid.

4. Immediately place in the freezer for 30 minutes to harden.

how to use Apply to clean, dry lips with your finger. Reapply as needed.

tip This doubles as a pretty and very light highlighter that looks beautiful underneath the arch of your eyebrow.

modification You can get creative with the color mica powder you use in this balm. Just make sure that the mica color you choose is safe for use on the lips—not all are!

* See page 18 for instructions.

new skin who dis setting spray

This setting spray keeps makeup in place all day long. Witch hazel is the magic maker: It shrinks pores! Coupled with lavender oil to naturally fight bacteria (which means fewer makeup-induced breakouts!), this setting spray is one your skin will love.

what you will need

- 4-oz (120-ml) spray bottle
- Funnel
- 1/3 cup (80 ml) rose water
- 1 tbsp (15 ml) witch hazel
- 1 tbsp (15 ml) aloe vera gel
- 10 drops lavender oil

MAKES ONE 4-OUNCE (120-ML) BOTTLE

step by step

1. Pour all the ingredients into the spray bottle using a funnel.

2. Shake well.

how to use Spray on your face after applying makeup. You can also use it throughout the day to refresh makeup—or use it as a pore-tightening spray without makeup.

"i dew" setting spray

This spray works best when used before and after applying makeup. The moisture-locking spray hydrates skin before makeup application. When applying the spray again after putting on your makeup, it keeps your look fresh and dewy regardless of how dry your environment is.

what you will need

- 4-oz (120-ml) spray bottle
- Funnel
- 1/3 cup (80 ml) rose water
- 2 tsp (10 ml) witch hazel
- 1 tbsp (15 ml) vegetable glycerin
- 1 tsp almond oil
- 1 tsp aloe vera gel
- 1 tsp fractionated coconut oil

MAKES ONE 4-OUNCE (120-ML) BOTTLE

step by step

1. Pour all the ingredients into the spray bottle using a funnel.

2. Shake well.

how to use Spray onto your face after applying makeup. You can also use it without makeup as a hydrating facial spray that shrinks pores.

tip Use this spray before and after makeup application to seal in your look with hydration.

shine bright like a diamond setting spray

Keep your makeup from moving all day . . . or all night . . . with this shimmery setting spray. The mica powder adds a subtle glow that puts your skin in the spotlight. Get ready to be the star of the show when the spotlight hits your skin.

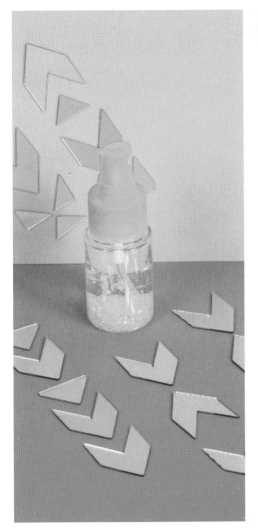

what you will need

- 4-oz (120-ml) spray bottle
- Funnel
- ⅓ cup (80 ml) rose water
- 1 tbsp (15 ml) witch hazel
- 1 tbsp (15 ml) vegetable glycerin
- ¼ tsp mica powder (iridescent)

MAKES ONE 4-OUNCE (120-ML) BOTTLE

step by step

1. Pour all the ingredients into the spray bottle using a funnel.
2. Shake well.

how to use Spray liberally onto your face after applying makeup. You can also use it on the neck and chest.

tip For an understated look, try using this setting spray sans makeup—or skip the foundation and focus on your brows, lashes, and lips and finish your look with this glow-enhancing spray.

modification Add 1 tsp of vitamin E oil to turn this setting spray into a hydrating and shimmery skin enhancer.

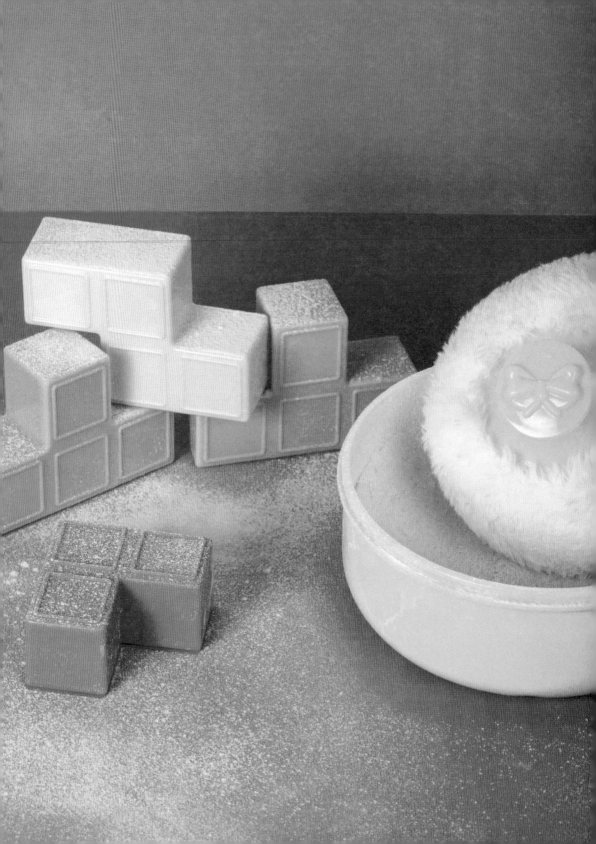

buildable beauty
setting powder

When it comes to setting your makeup and preventing shine, layering is key. To keep both in check, this setting powder is all that you need. Cornstarch, arrowroot powder, and silica form an oil-fighting trifecta. Use on a bare face to control oil and unwanted shine. Use over makeup to control shine and keep makeup from migrating. This powder is both buildable and sleek for an effortless matte finish any hour of the day.

what you will need

- 50-gram cosmetic container with sifter and lid
- 1 tsp cornstarch
- 2 tbsp (16 g) arrowroot powder
- 2 tsp silica
- Iron oxides (brown and yellow)

MAKES ONE 50-GRAM CONTAINER

step by step

1. Put the cornstarch, arrowroot powder, and silica in the cosmetic container. Put on the lid. Shake well to incorporate the ingredients. This will create a translucent setting powder. If you would like a tinted setting powder, continue to step 2:

2. Use a very small amount of brown and/or yellow iron oxides to change the color of the setting powder to match your skin tone.

  a. Start by putting a tiny amount of the brown iron oxide into the powder and shake well. Keep doing this until the powder matches your overall skin shade.

  b. If you have a pink or blue undertone, you may not need the yellow iron oxide. If your undertone is a bit yellow, you may need a pinch of the yellow iron oxide to make the powder blend seamlessly into your skin.

3. After you're done shaking the mixture, remove the lid and put the sifter back on the container. If there is some excess product that pushes its way through the holes on the sifter, you can discard this. Screw on the lid.

how to use Apply all over your face with a large fluffy brush to set makeup. It can also be used without makeup to control oil and shine.

tip If you have any oily areas on your face, apply a little extra setting powder to mop up the shine.

modification If you would like a tinted setting powder, you can alter the color of the powder by using different iron oxides than mentioned above. You can also use cocoa powder if you'd like a bit of a warmer tone to your powder.

liquid gold highlighter

This shimmery liquid can be used as a highlighter with or without makeup. That's not all that this super product can do, though. Try mixing in a few drops with your foundation for glow-boosted coverage. Drop some product in with your eye shadow for eyes that look like they're worth millions! Mix these drops with your lip gloss for the glossiest pout ever.

what you will need

- 30-ml bottle with dropper lid
- Funnel
- 2 tsp aloe vera gel
- ½ tsp argan oil
- ½ tsp pomegranate oil

- 10 drops vitamin E oil
- ¼ tsp magnesium stearate
- ½ tsp mica powder (iridescent)
- ½ tsp mica powder (bronze)

MAKES ONE 30-ML CONTAINER

step by step

1. Using a funnel, put the aloe vera gel, argan oil, pomegranate oil, and vitamin E oil in the bottle. Shake well to incorporate all the ingredients.

2. Put the magnesium stearate and mica powders into the bottle.

3. Shake well to incorporate all the ingredients.

It is normal for the ingredients to settle with time. Shake well before use.

how to use Use the dropper to apply the highlighter to a damp blending sponge. Blend onto the top of your cheekbones, temples, cupid's bow, inner corners of eyes, under the brow bone, or anywhere you want a beautiful glow.

tip You can use a couple of drops for a subtle glow, but that glow can be supercharged by adding even more drops.

modification You can modify your drops for different uses. Try iridescent mica powders for a face-highlighting drop. Try bronze and gold mica powders for drops you use near your eyes or in place of eye shadow. Try light pink mica powder (make sure it's safe for use in lip products) in your drops for a subtle flush for your lips.

slay all day highlighter

Throw this highlighter in your purse for an easy beauty-on-the-go solution. It quickly takes your look from day to night. Go from class to a girls' night out, or straight from work to date night. All you need is 60 seconds and this little pot of shimmer to get your glow on.

what you will need

- 50-gram glass cosmetic container with lid
- Double boiler*
- Funnel
- 1 tsp beeswax pellets

- 2 tbsp (30 ml) coconut oil
- ¼ tsp castor oil
- ¼ tsp vitamin E oil
- 1 tsp mica powder (iridescent)

MAKES ONE 50-GRAM CONTAINER

step by step

1. In a double boiler over medium heat, melt the beeswax pellets and coconut oil. Remove from the heat.

2. Add the castor oil and vitamin E oil. Stir well.

3. Add the mica powder. Stir well.

4. Using a funnel, transfer the mixture to the cosmetic container and carefully add the lid.

5. Immediately place the container in the freezer for 30 minutes to harden.

how to use Using your finger or a makeup sponge, apply this dewy salve to places on your face and body that you want to shine.

tip Start with a little bit and build from there. A little can go a long way! Use this highlighter under your brow bone and on the inner corners of your eyes for a subtle wide-eyed look.

modification Add 10 drops of any essential oil you love for a fragrance-infused highlighter with aromatherapy benefits. Looking to increase your glow? Double the amount of mica powder to use as a highlighter with super sparkle.

See page 18 for instructions.

shape-up brow pomade

For a perfectly polished arch, look no further than a pomade. A clear pomade is a great way to hold brows in place while also giving the illusion of a little extra volume. Looking to make more of an impact? Tint your pomade with iron oxides to bulk up your brows' natural beauty.

step by step

1. Melt the white beeswax pellets and coconut oil in a double boiler over medium heat. Remove from the heat.

2. Add the vegetable glycerin, jojoba oil, vitamin E oil, and castor oil to the melted beeswax. Stir until fully incorporated. If you want a clear brow pomade, skip to step 4.

3. Add the iron oxides to the mixture to match your brow color. For lighter hair, add the tiniest pinch (tiny!) of brown iron oxide. For brunettes, add ⅛ tsp of brown iron oxide. For raven-haired ladies, add ⅛ tsp of brown iron oxide and a teeny tiny pinch of black iron oxide. Stir until fully incorporated.

4. Using the funnel, pour the mixture into the cosmetic container and carefully add the lid.

5. Place immediately in the freezer for 30 minutes to harden.

how to use Dip angled brow brush into pomade and apply with upward and outward strokes.

tip For a different pomade look, try using a spoolie (a mascara wand/brow brush) to apply the pomade using upward and outward strokes.

modification Looking for a firmer hold? Skip adding the vegetable glycerin for a stickier formula.

* See page 18 for instructions.

what you will need

- 50-gram glass cosmetic container with lid
- Double boiler*
- Funnel
- 1 tsp white beeswax pellets
- 2 tbsp (30 ml) coconut oil
- ¼ tsp vegetable glycerin
- 5 drops jojoba oil
- 5 drops vitamin E oil
- ¼ tsp castor oil
- Iron oxides (brown and/or black)

MAKES ONE 50-GRAM CONTAINER

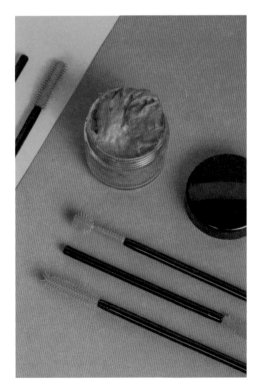

brows on fleek brow gel

Brows frame your face, so give them the attention that they deserve. The beauty of this brow gel is that it can be used with or without makeup. Brush brows into place for a polished and natural look. If you're feeling like getting dolled up, brush into place and allow the gel to set after applying a bold brow powder.

what you will need

- 10 ml mascara tube with wand
- Funnel
- 1 tbsp (15 ml) aloe vera gel
- 10 drops castor oil

MAKES ONE 10 ML TUBE

step by step

1. In a small dish, mix the aloe vera gel and castor oil until incorporated.

2. Use the funnel to transfer the mixture to the mascara tube.

3. Screw the wand lid on tightly.

how to use Use the gel to brush brows upward and then outward to hold brow hairs in place. If you are using brow makeup in addition to this gel, apply gel and wait 3 minutes before applying brow powder.

tip This brow gel holds hair in place all day. It can also be used on baby hairs around your hairline to keep flyaways in place.

crush on my blush

This light-pink blush is the perfect shade for a natural daytime look. Think sugar, bubblegum, and Candy Crush. This shade looks beautiful on natural skin or partnered with bronzer for a Malibu Beach babe look.

what you will need

- 50-gram cosmetic container with sifter and lid
- 1 tbsp (8 g) arrowroot powder
- 2 tsp silica
- 2 tsp hibiscus powder
- ¼ tsp mica powder (light pink)

ONE 50-GRAM CONTAINER

step by step

1. Put the arrowroot powder and silica into the cosmetic container. Put on the lid and shake well.

2. Take off the lid. Add the hibiscus powder and mica powder. Put on the lid and shake well.

3. After you're done shaking the mixture, remove the lid and put the sifter back on the container. If there is some excess product that pushes its way through the holes on the sifter, you can discard this. Screw on the lid.

how to use Using a blush brush or a fluffy brush, apply the blush to the apples of your cheeks.

tip Start with a little bit of blush and build from there. Blush is meant to accentuate, not take center stage. A little goes a long way.

orange popsicle cream blush

This blush will transport you to an ice cream stand on the pier by the ocean. The light orange is subtle and sweet—just like your favorite childhood treats. This light color with its subtle shimmer works on eyes, cheeks, and lips, so you can throw this in your beach bag and be ready for whatever the day brings.

what you will need

- 50-gram glass cosmetic container with lid
- Double boiler*
- Funnel
- 1 tbsp (15 ml) coconut oil
- 1 tbsp (15 g) shea butter

- ½ tbsp vegetable emulsifying wax
- ½ tbsp aloe vera gel
- ½ tsp turmeric
- ¼ tsp iron oxide (red)
- ¼ tsp mica powder (gold)

MAKES ONE 50-GRAM CONTAINER

step by step

1. Melt the coconut oil, shea butter, and vegetable emulsifying wax in a double boiler over medium heat. Remove from the heat.

2. Add the aloe vera gel to the mixture. Stir until fully incorporated.

3. Add the turmeric, iron oxide, and mica powder. Stir well until fully incorporated.

4. Use a funnel to put the mixture in the cosmetic container and carefully add the lid.

5. Immediately put the mixture in the freezer for 30 minutes to harden.

how to use Apply to the apples of your cheeks using your fingers. Blend well.

tip Apply this cream blush higher on the apples of your cheeks, closer to your temples, for an instant perk-up. Try using it without any other makeup for a subtle flush of color.

modification Double the amount of mica powder for a beautiful cream eye shadow. It also works as a highlighter! If you would like a more intense shade, increase the amount of red iron oxide and turmeric.

* See page 18 for instructions.

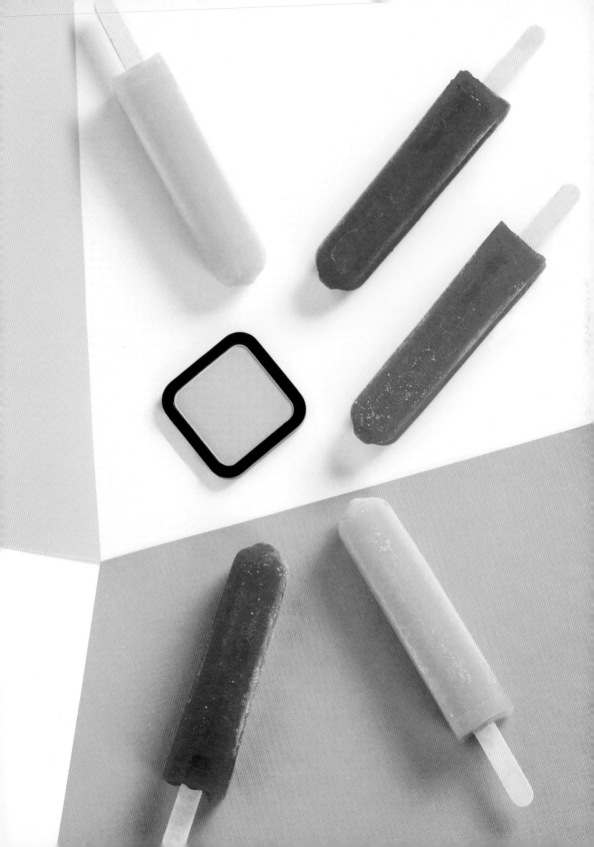

boss babe powder blush

This reddish-brown rouge means business. You can use this color to dress up a casual look or wear it to work for the bossiest blush. The rust hue pairs perfectly with winged liner and a matte lip.

what you will need

- 50-gram cosmetic container with sifter and lid
- 1 tbsp (8 g) arrowroot powder
- 2 tsp silica
- ½ tsp iron oxide (red)
- 1 tsp cocoa powder
- ¼ tsp mica powder (bronze)

MAKES ONE 50-GRAM CONTAINER

step by step

1. Put the arrowroot powder and silica into the cosmetic container. Put on the lid and shake well.

2. Take off the lid. Add the iron oxide, cocoa powder, and mica powder. Put on the lid and shake well.

3. After you're done shaking the mixture, remove the lid and put the sifter back on the container. If there is some excess product that pushes its way through the holes on the sifter, you can discard this. Screw on the lid.

how to use Using a blush brush or a fluffy brush, apply the blush to the apples of your cheeks.

tip Start with a little bit of blush and build from there. Blush is meant to accentuate.

pretty in pink cream blush

This is the kind of blush you would see coupled with a pair of oversize shades.

what you will need

- 50-gram glass cosmetic container with lid
- Double boiler*
- Funnel
- 1 tbsp (15 ml) coconut oil
- 1 tbsp (15 g) shea butter
- ½ tbsp vegetable emulsifying wax
- ½ tbsp aloe vera gel
- 1 tsp beetroot powder
- 1 tsp hibiscus powder
- ¼ tsp mica powder (pink)

MAKES ONE 50-GRAM CONTAINER

See page 18 for instructions.

step by step

1. Melt the coconut oil, shea butter, and vegetable emulsifying wax in a double boiler over medium heat. Remove from the heat.

2. Add the aloe vera gel to the mixture. Stir until fully incorporated.

3. Add the beetroot powder, hibiscus owder, and mica powder. Stir well until fully incorporated.

4. Use a funnel to put the mixture in the cosmetic container and carefully add the lid.

5. Immediately put the mixture in the freezer for 30 minutes to harden.

how to use Apply to the apples of your cheeks using your fingers. Blend well.

ruby renegade powder rouge

This rouge is perfect for those days when you want to take the world by storm. The deep-red blush is flashy. Apply lightly with a large fluffy blush for a subtle effect. Apply with a dense blush brush for a bold pop of color.

what you will need

- 50-gram cosmetic container with sifter and lid
- 1 tbsp (8 g) arrowroot powder

- 2 tsp silica
- 1 tsp iron oxide (red)
- ¼ tsp mica powder (bronze)

MAKES ONE 50-GRAM CONTAINER

step by step

1. Put the arrowroot powder and silica into the cosmetic container. Put on the lid and shake well.

2. Take off the lid. Add the iron oxide and mica powder. Put on the lid and shake well.

3. After you're done shaking the mixture, remove the lid and put the sifter back on the container. If there is some excess product that pushes its way through the holes on the sifter, you can discard this. Screw on the lid.

how to use Using a blush brush or a fluffy brush, apply the blush to the apples of your cheeks.

tip Try applying a very light dusting of blush in the direct center of the apples of your cheeks for a subtle effect that appears youthful and natural.

modification If you want to make a major statement, double the amount of iron oxide to give this rouge some extra oomph. You can also remove the mica powder for a matte blush look with major attitude.

fresh face primer

A face primer is the key to getting makeup to stay put as you go about your day. This primer is ultra-hydrating and also keeps makeup-migrating oil at bay. Rose water and aloe vera gel keep the pH in balance and hydrate the skin.

what you will need

- 3-oz (90-ml) silicone squeeze bottle
- Funnel
- 1 tbsp (15 ml) rose water
- 1 tbsp (15 ml) vegetable glycerin
- 5 tbsp (75 ml) aloe vera gel
- ¼ tsp almond oil
- ¼ tsp jojoba oil
- ¼ tsp vitamin E oil

MAKES ONE 3-OUNCE (90-ML) BOTTLE

step by step

1. Put all the ingredients into a mixing bowl. Stir well with a whisk to fully incorporate.

2. Using a funnel, transfer the mixture to the squeeze bottle.

how to use Apply after moisturizing, but before applying foundation. Give the primer about 60 seconds to dry before applying makeup.

tip If you're looking to control oil production and keep your face hydrated, you can use this primer without makeup to keep your skin under control.

modification If you're looking for a dewier primer, double the amount of aloe vera gel.

perfect pout lip primer

This lip primer hydrates lips and perfects every crease, helping you achieve your #lipgoals. Ingredients like castor oil and beeswax help deeply hydrate your lips for a flawless finish!

what you will need

- 50-gram glass cosmetic container with lid
- Double boiler*
- 1 tbsp (15 g) white beeswax pellets
- 3 tbsp (45 ml) castor oil
- 1 tsp vitamin E oil

MAKES ONE 50-GRAM CONTAINER

step by step

1. In a double boiler over medium heat, melt the white beeswax pellets completely. Remove from the heat.

2. While the beeswax is still warm and melted, add the castor oil and vitamin E oil. Stir well to fully incorporate.

3. Transfer the mixture to the cosmetic container and carefully add the lid. Place in the freezer for 30 minutes to harden.

how to use Apply to clean, dry lips before applying lip color or lip gloss to help the color hold.

tip This primer is ultra effective if you use it after a lip scrub.

See page 18 for instructions.

eyes don't stray eye primer

If you are going to take the time to carefully apply some eye shadow to your lids, take the extra step to help that shadow stay put. For major staying power (and built-in protection from the sun!), apply this to lids before applying shadow.

what you will need

- 50-gram glass cosmetic container with lid
- Double boiler*
- 2 tbsp (30 g) white beeswax pellets
- 2 tbsp (30 ml) aloe vera gel
- ½ tsp jojoba oil

- ½ tsp argan oil
- ½ tsp zinc oxide
- ½ tsp kaolin clay
- ½ tsp arrowroot powder

MAKES ONE 50-GRAM CONTAINER

step by step

1. Using a double boiler over medium heat, heat the white beeswax pellets, aloe vera gel, jojoba oil, and argan oil over medium heat until melted completely. While the mixture is melting, proceed to step 2.

2. In a small mixing bowl, whisk together the zinc oxide, kaolin clay, and arrowroot powder.

3. When the mixture from step 1 is completely melted and in the double boiler, add the dry mixture from step 2.

4. Work quickly and whisk the mixture until fully incorporated.*

5. Transfer the mixture to the cosmetic container and carefully add the lid. Place in the freezer for 30 minutes to harden.

how to use Apply to clean, dry eyelids before applying eye shadow or eye shimmer.

tip The zinc oxide in this primer acts as natural sun protection for your sensitive lids. This is a quick way to use your beauty routine to help save your skin.

modification If you are looking for a whiter base primer (to make bold shadow colors pop), double the amount of kaolin clay.

* See page 18 for instructions.

* If the mixture begins to harden too quickly, just heat in the double boiler and stir until fully incorporated.

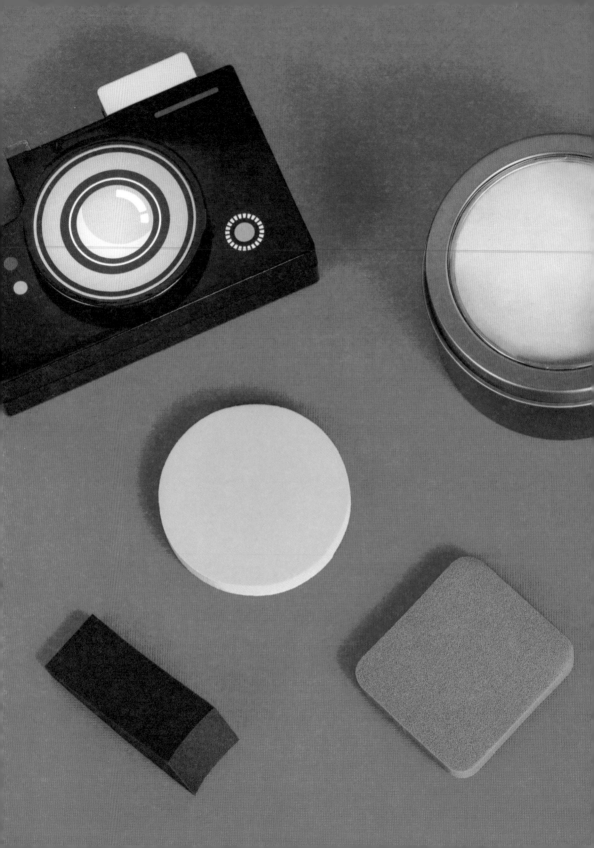

lookin' good for the press
powder foundation

The convenience of pressed powder in a compact (throw it in your purse or gym bag!) is unrivaled. Perfect to touch up on the go or if you're just looking for a little more coverage. Look pulled together in an instant with this pressed-powder foundation.

MAKEUP

what you will need

- Cosmetic compact
- Parchment paper
- Tamping tool
- 1 tbsp (8 g) arrowroot powder
- ¼ tsp silica
- ¼ tsp magnesium stearate
- ⅛ tsp zinc oxide

- ⅛ tsp kaolin clay
- ⅛ tsp mica powder (iridescent)
- Cocoa powder (amount varies, see step 2)
- Brown iron oxide (amount varies, see step 2)
- Yellow iron oxide (amount varies, see step 2)
- Jojoba oil (amount varies, see step 3)

MAKES ONE OR TWO COSMETIC COMPACTS

step by step

1. Add the arrowroot powder, silica, magnesium stearate, zinc oxide, kaolin clay, and mica powder to a mixing bowl. Mix well with a whisk.

2. Add the cocoa powder and iron oxides a little bit at a time, whisking to incorporate, until the powder is a good match for your skin tone. The best way to check is to brush it along your jawline to ensure that it blends in.

3. Add the jojoba oil 20 drops at a time. Mix well with a whisk. Keep doing this until the powder forms a chunky, crumbly "dough" (resembling a bunch of tiny pebbles).

4. Transfer part of the mixture to the cosmetic compact. Cover with parchment paper and use the tamping tool on top of the parchment paper to press down the mixture until there is a thin, flat layer.

5. Keep repeating this process until you have used up all of the mixture or your compact is full. Discard the excess (unless there is enough to fill another compact—then you can make two).

6. Leave the compact open for 24 hours to dry.

how to use After applying a facial primer, use a fluffy foundation brush, a kabuki brush, a makeup sponge, or a powder puff to apply this all over your face.

tip If you want a natural look, apply only a little bit of this foundation to the areas where your skin is a bit discolored or blemished and leave the rest of your skin bare.

modification If you're looking for a light-reflecting foundation to make you look "awake," double the amount of mica powder for a more radiant effect.

no im-pore-fections powder foundation

This soft mineral powder foundation provides light coverage to blur slight imperfections. The zinc oxide provides natural sun protection while jojoba oil adds a hydrating effect to this powder. You can use a large fluffy brush for overall light coverage or a kabuki brush for more concentrated coverage.

what you will need

- 50-gram cosmetic container with sifter and lid
- 1 tbsp (8 g) arrowroot powder
- ¼ tsp silica
- ¼ tsp zinc oxide
- ¼ tsp kaolin clay
- ⅛ tsp mica powder (iridescent)
- 10 drops jojoba oil
- Cocoa powder (amount varies, see step 3)
- Brown iron oxide (amount varies, see step 3)
- Yellow iron oxide (amount varies, see step 3)

MAKES ONE 50-GRAM CONTAINER

step by step

1. Add the arrowroot powder, silica, zinc oxide, kaolin clay, and mica powder to a mixing bowl. Mix well with a whisk.

2. Add the jojoba oil. Mix well with a whisk.

3. Add the cocoa powder and iron oxides a little bit at a time, whisking to incorporate, until the powder is a good match for your skin tone. The best way to check is to brush it along your jawline and to ensure that it blends in.

4. Transfer the mixture to the cosmetic container. Affix the sifter and screw on the lid.

how to use After applying your facial primer, use a foundation brush or a kabuki brush to apply this powder all over your face.

tip Blend down from your jawline onto your neck to avoid any harsh makeup lines.

modification Would you like lighter coverage? Decrease the amount of zinc oxide and kaolin clay. Heavier coverage? Increase the amounts of those ingredients.

all about eyes eyeliner

This liner looks great on brown eyes—and it also brings out baby blues and highlights emerald green. This liner is a soft and natural go-to for your daytime liner look.

what you will need

- 50-gram glass cosmetic container with lid
- Double boiler*
- 1 tbsp (15 ml) coconut oil
- 1 tbsp (15 g) shea butter
- 2 tsp cocoa powder

MAKES ONE 50-GRAM CONTAINER

step by step

1. In a double boiler over medium heat, completely melt the coconut oil and shea butter. Remove from the heat.

2. Add the cocoa powder and whisk until completely incorporated.

3. Transfer the mixture to the cosmetic container and carefully add the lid. Place immediately in the freezer for 30 minutes to harden.

how to use Use an angled eyeliner brush to line your lids.

tip Practice makes perfect. Try lining your top lid. Then try lining just the outer section of your top lid.

* See page 18 for instructions.

i'm not flirting with you mascara

They might think you're batting your eyelashes at them, but you know the truth: this mascara shows off your eyes and makes you the center of attention—whether you realize it or not!

what you will need

- 10-ml glass mascara container with eyelash/ eyebrow wand
- Double boiler*
- Small pipette
- ¼ tsp coconut oil
- ¼ tsp vitamin E oil
- ¼ tsp white beeswax pellets
- ¾ tsp aloe vera gel
- ½ tsp activated charcoal

MAKES ONE 10-ML CONTAINER

* See page 18 for instructions.

step by step

1. Heat the coconut oil, vitamin E oil, and white beeswax pellets in a double boiler over medium heat until completely melted. Remove from the heat.

2. Add the aloe vera gel and activated charcoal. Stir until fully incorporated.

3. Using a small pipette, transfer to the mascara container and carefully add the lid.

how to use Using the mascara wand, brush mascara onto clean, dry lashes in an upward and outward motion.

cat cream eyeliner

Black liner has been a staple since makeup was invented. It has long signified beauty, strength, and power. A bold line communicates the same message today. Channel your inner queen and make Cleopatra proud.

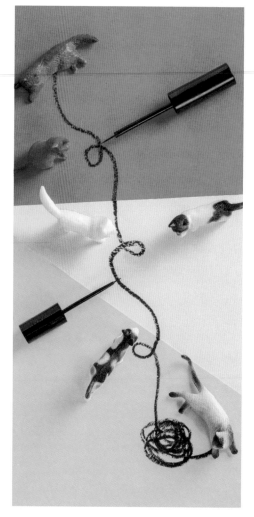

what you will need

- **50-gram glass cosmetic container with lid**
- **Double boiler***
- **1 tbsp (15 ml) coconut oil**
- **1 tbsp (15 g) shea butter**
- **2 tsp activated charcoal**

MAKES ONE 50-GRAM CONTAINER

step by step

1. In a double boiler over medium heat, completely melt the coconut oil and shea butter. Remove from the heat.

2. Add the activated charcoal and whisk until completely incorporated.

3. Transfer the mixture to the cosmetic container and carefully add the lid. Place immediately place in the freezer for 30 minutes to harden.

how to use Use an angled eyeliner brush to apply the liner around your eyes.

tip This liner looks beautiful when drawn into a tiny wing at the corner of the eye.

modification Want a fun party liner? Add ½ tsp of iridescent mica powder to this recipe for a party-perfect look.

See page 18 for instructions.

warrior makeup remover

After a long day battling life's ups and downs, you deserve a quick-and-easy way to revive yourself. Keep these makeup remover wipes next to your bed for the perfect solution to taking off your cosmetics at night. The coconut oil is strong enough to break down waterproof makeup, but gentle enough to be used around the eyes. The ingredients are hydrating and the perfect way to help your skin wind down so that it can recharge for tomorrow.

step by step

1. Gently heat the rose water in a saucepan over low heat. When hot, remove the pan from the heat.

2. Add the fractionated coconut oil and aloe vera gel to the water. Stir well until fully incorporated.

3. Add the coconut milk. Stir until fully incorporated.

4. Add the witch hazel, jojoba oil, and lavender oil. Stir until fully incorporated.

5. Put as many cotton rounds in the jar as will fit.

6. Using the funnel, slowly pour the mixture over the cotton rounds. Pause occasionally to allow the cotton rounds to absorb the mixture before pouring again.

7. Ensure that the cotton rounds are fully saturated. Screw on the lid.

how to use Use to remove makeup on the face and neck. Take care around the eyes.

tip The lavender oil acts as a natural antibacterial agent, helping to preserve the makeup remover wipes and stop acne.

modification Looking for a luxurious way to have these makeup remover wipes double as a skin treatment? Add a few drops of vitamin E oil and jasmine oil in step 4 for a hydrating and skin-softening way to remove makeup.

what you will need

- 8-oz (240-ml) glass jar with lid
- Cotton rounds
- Funnel
- 2 tbsp (30 ml) rose water
- 1 tbsp (15 ml) fractionated coconut oil
- 2 tbsp (30 ml) aloe vera gel
- 2 tbsp (30 ml) coconut milk
- 1 tbsp (15 ml) witch hazel
- ¼ tsp jojoba oil
- 30 drops lavender oil

MAKES ONE 8-OUNCE (240-ML) JAR

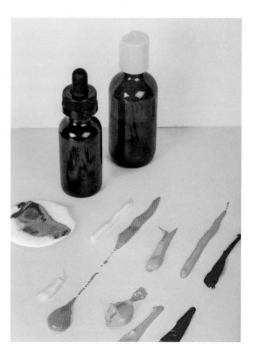

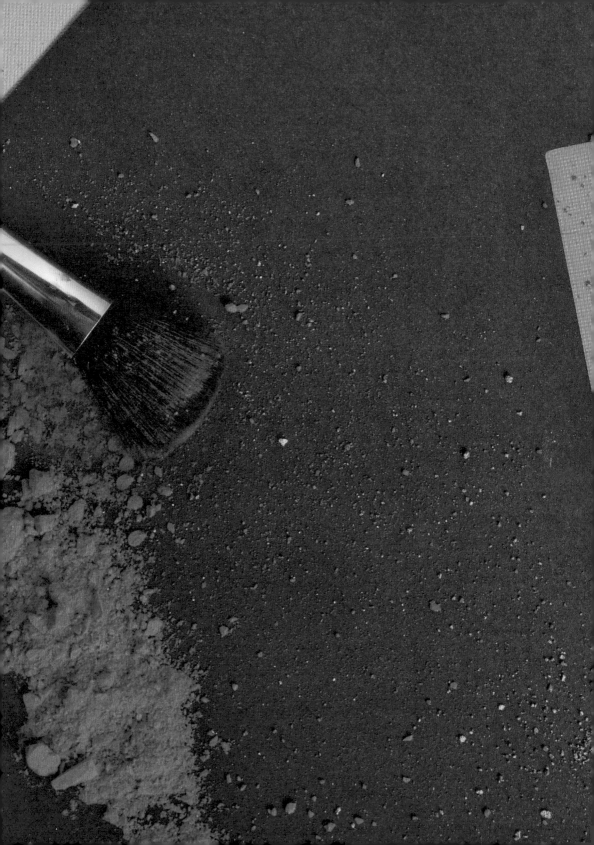

EYE SHADOWS

Eyes are windows into the soul, and eye shadow can quickly transform you into a confident queen, with gorgeous and enticing color blends and combos. The great thing about eye shadow is that you can build and customize it however you like. Simply apply and let your personality shine through. Each color can be made either as a powder or a cream, so the eye's the limit!

truly timeless
powder eye shadow

If there's one eye shadow color that's always in style, it's shimmery white. It's a great "go to" shade that creates a base for the rest of your lid. Although it may be simple, you can be sure this eye shadow will stand the test of time.

what you will need

- Six 3-ml cosmetic containers with lids
- 1 tsp arrowroot powder
- ¼ tsp silica
- 1 tsp kaolin clay
- ¼ tsp mica powder (iridescent)

- 5 drops rosehip oil
- 5 drops vitamin E oil
- 5 drops pomegranate oil

MAKES SIX 3-ML COSMETIC CONTAINERS

step by step

1. In a small mixing bowl, whisk together the arrowroot powder, silica, kaolin clay, and mica powder.

2. Add the rosehip oil, vitamin E oil, and pomegranate oil. Whisk together until fully incorporated.

3. Transfer the eye shadow to the cosmetic containers.

how to use Using an eye shadow brush (or even your finger), apply shadow to lids.

tip Use this bright white shadow on the inner corners of your eyes for a bright-eyed look. Apply a tiny amount of this shimmery shadow to your cupid's bow—the area right above the center of your upper lip—for a beautiful enhancement.

modification Increase the amount of kaolin clay for a brighter white. Also, add as much mica powder as you like. Remember: the more mica, the more sparkle!

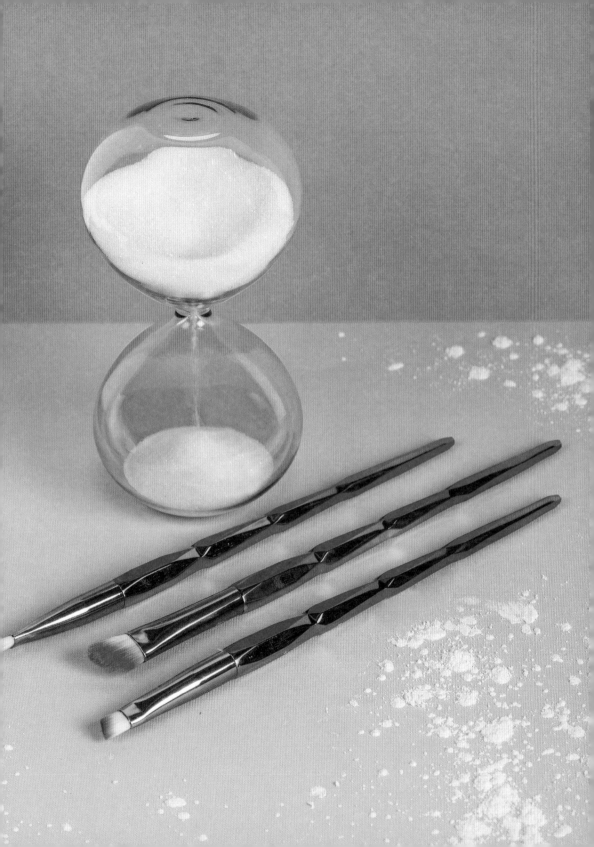

snow queen
cream eye shadow

You'll feel like the Queen of Winter in this fabulous, frosty shadow. It's luminous color, when applied to the corners of your eyes, is like a dusting of snow. It also looks stunning when applied across the lid and up to the brow bone.

what you will need

- Six 3-ml glass cosmetic containers with lids
- Double boiler*
- Pipette
- ½ tsp avocado butter
- ½ tsp cocoa butter
- 1 tsp vegetable emulsifying wax
- ⅛ tsp magnesium stearate

- 1 tbsp (15 ml) aloe vera gel
- 10 drops rosehip oil
- 5 drops vitamin E oil
- 5 drops pomegranate oil
- ⅛ tsp arrowroot powder
- ¼ tsp mica powder (iridescent)
- ¾ tsp kaolin clay

MAKES SIX 3-ML COSMETIC CONTAINERS

step by step

1. In a double boiler over medium heat, completely melt the avocado butter, cocoa butter, and vegetable emulsifying wax.

2. Add the magnesium stearate while the mixture is still over the heat. Stir until completely incorporated. Remove from the heat.

3. While mixture is still warm and melted, add the aloe vera gel, rosehip oil, vitamin E oil, and pomegranate oil. Stir until completely incorporated.

4. While the mixture is still warm and melted, add the arrowroot powder, mica powder, and kaolin clay. Stir until completely incorporated.

5. Transfer the mixture to the cosmetic containers using a pipette and carefully add the lid.

6. Wait at least 60 minutes for the eye shadow to harden.

how to use Apply to clean, dry eyelids (or eyelids that have been prepped with eye shadow primer) using your finger. Blend well.

tip Apply to the inner corners of your eyes and underneath your brow bone for an instant boost.

modification Omit the mica powder for a matte base shadow that can be used alone or as a primer.

* See page 18 for instructions.

not-so-basic beige powder eye shadow

This beige shadow looks chic and understated when worn alone. It is also an incredibly versatile shade—pair it with a darker color in the crease for eyes that pop. Couple it with a bright color for an unexpected combination. Your imagination is the only limit when it comes to applying for this not-so-basic beige.

what you will need

- Six 3-ml glass cosmetic containers with lids
- 1 tsp arrowroot powder
- ¼ tsp silica
- ½ tsp kaolin clay
- ½ tsp cocoa powder

- ¼ tsp mica powder (iridescent)
- 5 drops rosehip oil
- 5 drops vitamin E oil
- 5 drops pomegranate oil

MAKES SIX 3-ML COSMETIC CONTAINERS

step by step

1. In a small mixing bowl, whisk together the arrowroot powder, silica, kaolin clay, cocoa powder, and mica powder.

2. Add the rosehip oil, vitamin E oil, and pomegranate oil. Whisk together until fully incorporated.

3. Transfer the eye shadow to the cosmetic containers.

how to use Using an eye shadow brush (or even your finger!), apply shadow to lids.

tip This color is a great everyday shade and is a beautiful neutral that can act as a base for endless eye shadow looks.

modification Amp up the shimmer and double the amount of mica powder for the ultimate nighttime neutral. Want a lighter shade? Increase the amount of kaolin clay. Want a darker shade? Increase the amount of cocoa powder. Want a matte shadow? Don't use mica powder.

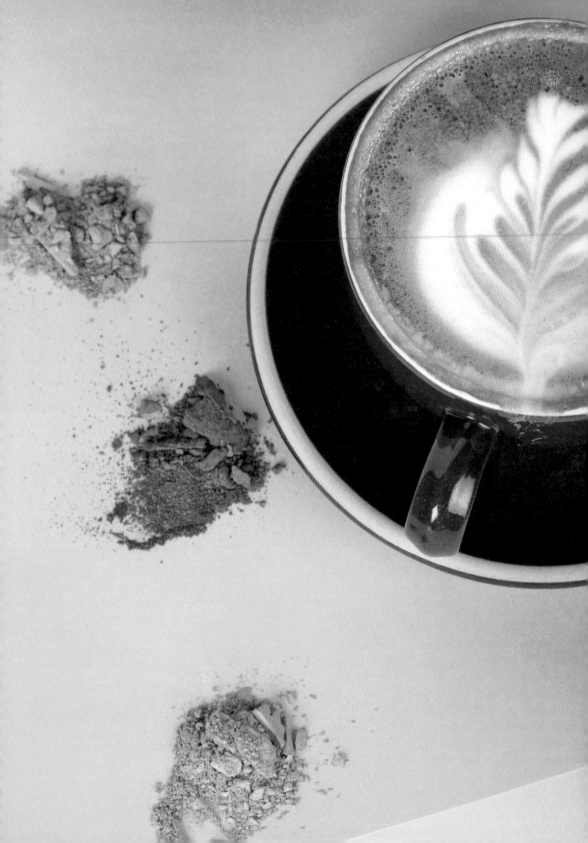

cafe au lait beige cream eye shadow

This coffee-and-cream-hued eye shadow is perfect for working the day away at your local coffee shop. It's subtle brown tint, delicious mocha fragrance, and shimmer of iridescent mica powder will pump you up more than a caramel macchiato.

what you will need

- Six 3-ml glass cosmetic containers with lids
- Double boiler*
- Pipette
- ½ tsp avocado butter
- ½ tsp cocoa butter
- 1 tsp vegetable emulsifying wax
- ⅛ tsp magnesium stearate
- 1 tbsp (15 ml) aloe vera gel

- 10 drops rosehip oil
- 5 drops vitamin E oil
- 5 drops pomegranate oil
- ⅛ tsp arrowroot powder
- ½ tsp kaolin clay
- ¼ tsp mica powder (iridescent)
- ¼ tsp cocoa powder

MAKES SIX 3-ML COSMETIC CONTAINERS

step by step

1. In a double boiler over medium heat, completely melt the avocado butter, cocoa butter, and vegetable emulsifying wax.

2. Add the magnesium stearate while the mixture is still over the heat. Stir until completely incorporated. Remove from the heat.

3. While the mixture is still warm and melted, add the aloe vera gel, rosehip oil, vitamin E oil, and pomegranate oil. Stir until completely incorporated.

4. While the mixture is still warm and melted, add the arrowroot powder, kaolin clay, mica powder, and cocoa powder. Stir until completely incorporated.

5. Transfer the mixture to the cosmetic containers using a pipette and carefully add the lid.

6. Wait at least 60 minutes for the eye shadow to harden.

how to use Apply to clean, dry eyelids (or eyelids that have been prepped with eye shadow primer) using your finger. Blend well.

tip Looking for a fail-safe neutral? This shadow is it. This shade is great for beginners because it's light and blendable. Perfect your cream eye shadow techniques with this shade first!

modification You can double the amount of vitamin E oil and turn this formula into a creamy nude lip balm.

* See page 18 for instructions.

black mamba powder eye shadow

Beware: Although this eyeshadow isn't venomous, one well-executed side eye will strike fear into the hearts of anyone who dares to hiss at you.

what you will need

- Six 3-ml cosmetic containers with lids
- 1 tsp arrowroot powder
- ¼ tsp silica
- ½ tsp iron oxide (black)
- ¼ tsp mica powder (iridescent)
- 5 drops rosehip oil
- 5 drops vitamin E oil
- 5 drops pomegranate oil

MAKES SIX 3-ML COSMETIC CONTAINERS

step by step

1. In a small mixing bowl, whisk together the arrowroot powder, silica, iron oxide, and mica powder.

2. Add the rosehip oil, vitamin E oil, and pomegranate oil. Whisk together until fully incorporated.

3. Transfer the eye shadow to the cosmetic containers.

how to use Using an eye shadow brush (or even your finger), apply shadow to lids.

tip A little goes a long way. Use this dark shadow to accent eyes. Really want to go for it? Cover the whole upper lid in this shadow and use a shadow brush to apply along your lower lash line for an intense look. This shadow can also double as an eyeliner. Simply take an angled eyeliner brush, slightly dampen it, and dip it into the shadow. Use the brush to press on your newly created "liquid eyeliner."

modification Omit the iridescent mica powder for a matte black shadow. Or, make it even darker by adding more black iron oxide.

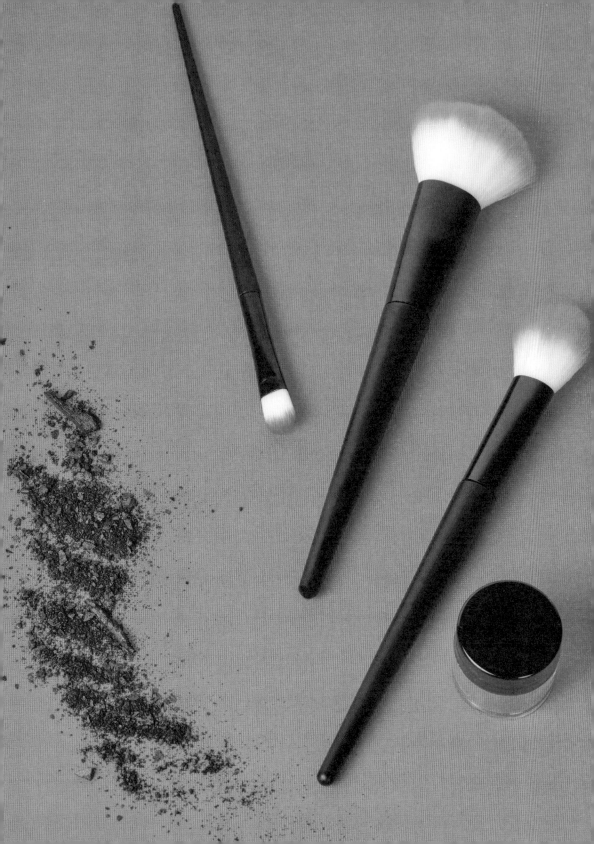

make a wish
cream eye shadow

This shadow will remind you of the deep, dark color at the bottom of a wishing well. No need to wish for enticing eyes, though. This creamy concoction will take care of that!

what you will need

- Six 3-ml glass cosmetic container with lids
- Double boiler*
- Pipette
- ½ tsp avocado butter
- ½ tsp cocoa butter
- 1 tsp vegetable emulsifying wax
- ⅛ tsp magnesium stearate

- 1 tbsp (15 ml) aloe vera gel
- 10 drops rosehip oil
- 5 drops vitamin E oil
- 5 drops pomegranate oil
- ⅛ tsp arrowroot powder
- ¼ tsp mica powder (iridescent)
- ¾ tsp iron oxide (black)

MAKES SIX 3-ML COSMETIC CONTAINERS

step by step

1. In a double boiler over medium heat, completely melt the avocado butter, cocoa butter, and vegetable emulsifying wax.

2. Add the magnesium stearate while the mixture is still over the heat. Stir until completely incorporated. Remove from the heat.

3. While the mixture is still warm and melted, add the aloe vera gel, rosehip oil, vitamin E oil, and pomegranate oil. Stir until completely incorporated.

4. While the mixture is still warm and melted, add the arrowroot powder, mica powder, and iron oxide. Stir until completely incorporated.

5. Transfer the mixture to the cosmetic containers using a pipette and carefully add the lid.

6. Wait at least 60 minutes for the eye shadow to harden.

how to use Apply to clean, dry eyelids (or eyelids that have been prepped with eye shadow primer) using your finger. Blend well.

tip You can use this eye shadow on the entire eyelid and all around the eye for a sultry effect.

modification Double the amount of mica powder for a wishing well full of stars.

* See page 18 for instructions.

silver stunner
powder eye shadow

Cloudy day? No problem. Brighten your spirit while you brighten your lids. This vibrant shadow will have you singin' in the rain in no time!

what you will need

- Six 3-ml cosmetic containers with lids
- 1 tsp arrowroot powder
- ¼ tsp silica
- ½ tsp kaolin clay
- ¼ tsp iron oxide (black)
- ¼ tsp mica powder (silver)
- 5 drops rosehip oil
- 5 drops vitamin E oil
- 5 drops pomegranate oil

MAKES SIX 3-ML COSMETIC CONTAINERS

step by step

1. In a small mixing bowl, whisk together the arrowroot powder, silica, kaolin clay, iron oxide, and mica powder.

2. Add the rosehip oil, vitamin E oil, and pomegranate oil. Whisk together until fully incorporated.

3. Transfer the eye shadow to the cosmetic containers.

how to Use Using an eye shadow brush (or your finger), apply shadow to lids.

tip This shadow can be applied wet or dry. Try putting it on your lid with a damp fingertip for a bold look. Try applying this shadow to the upper lid and all the way around the eye before applying mascara on both the top and bottom lashes. This gray color will make all eye colors pop.

modification You can swap out the silver mica powder for an iridescent mica for a softer effect. Or you can remove the mica powder for a moody, matte gray color instead, perfect for winter looks.

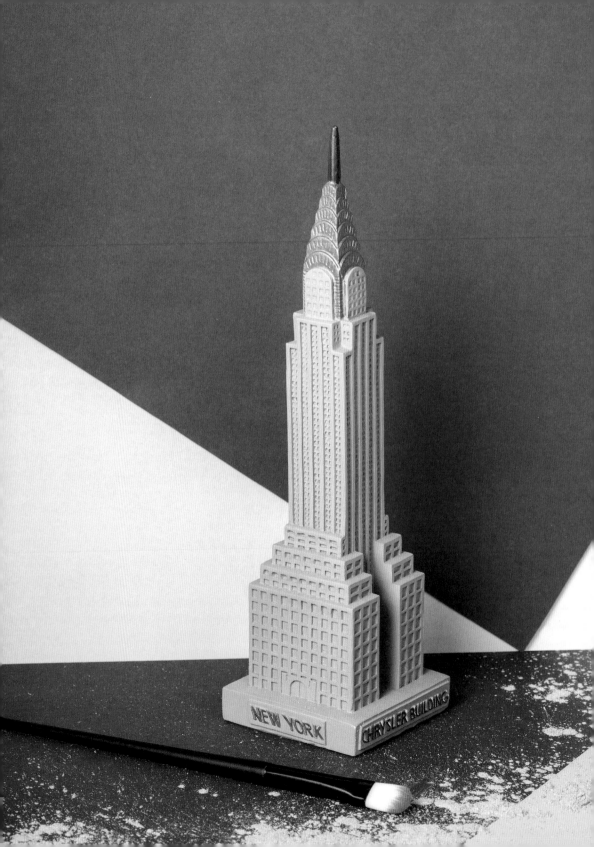

tower of power silver cream eye shadow

For days when you're feeling beaten down, try this gray eye shadow with metallic shine. This stormy steel shade is perfect to let the world know that you're tough as nails.

what you will need

- Six 3-ml glass cosmetic containers with lids
- Double boiler*
- Pipette
- ½ tsp avocado butter
- ½ tsp cocoa butter
- 1 tsp vegetable emulsifying wax
- ⅛ tsp magnesium stearate
- 1 tbsp (15 ml) aloe vera gel

- 10 drops rosehip oil
- 5 drops vitamin E oil
- 5 drops pomegranate oil
- ⅛ tsp arrowroot powder
- ¼ tsp mica powder (silver)
- ½ tsp iron oxide (black)
- ¼ tsp kaolin clay

MAKES SIX 3-ML COSMETIC CONTAINERS

step by step

1. In a double boiler over medium heat, completely melt the avocado butter, cocoa butter, and vegetable emulsifying wax.

2. Add the magnesium stearate while the mixture is still over the heat. Stir until completely incorporated. Remove from the heat.

3. While the mixture is still warm and melted, add the aloe vera gel, rosehip oil, vitamin E oil, and pomegranate oil. Stir until completely incorporated.

4. While the mixture is still warm and melted, add the arrowroot powder, mica powder, iron oxide, and kaolin clay. Stir until completely incorporated.

5. Transfer the mixture to the cosmetic containers using a pipette and carefully add the lid.

6. Wait at least 60 minutes for the eye shadow to harden.

how to use Apply to clean, dry eyelids (or eyelids that have been prepped with eye shadow primer) using your finger. Blend well.

tip Try wearing this on the inner corners of your eyes for an unexpectedly soft impact.

modification Add three times the amount of silver mica powder for an eye-catching lid topper.

* See page 18 for instructions.

"no bug"
powder eye shadow

This gorgeous metallic blue shimmer is so smooth and natural you'll hardly realize it's covering your lids. (But that won't stop everyone else from noticing it!)

what you will need

- Six 3-ml cosmetic containers with lids
- 1 tsp arrowroot powder
- ¼ tsp silica
- ¼ tsp kaolin clay
- 1 tsp mica powder (blue)
- ¼ tsp mica powder (gold)
- 5 drops rosehip oil
- 5 drops vitamin E oil
- 5 drops pomegranate oil

MAKES SIX 3-ML COSMETIC CONTAINERS

step by step

1. In a small mixing bowl, whisk together the arrowroot powder, silica, kaolin clay, and mica powders.

2. Add the rosehip oil, vitamin E oil, and pomegranate oil. Whisk together until fully incorporated.

3. Transfer the eye shadow to the cosmetic containers.

how to use Using an eye shadow brush (or even your finger), apply shadow to lids.

tip Instead of putting the shadow on your entire lid, use this blue eye shadow to make a subtle impact. Try using it in your crease or the outer corner of your eye for a daytime look. A little bit of color goes a long way. A colorful dot of blue on the inner corner of the eye really pops against an otherwise neutral look.

modification Add iridescent mica powder and turquoise mica to this shadow for a fun mermaid-like look. Or add iridescent mica powder instead of gold mica for a cosmic effect.

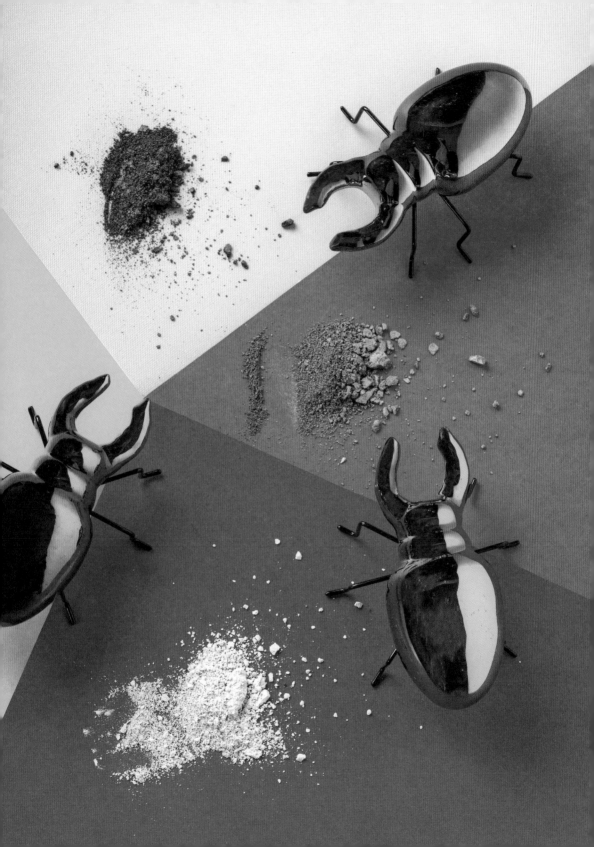

aquamarine
cream eye shadow

This vibrant eye shadow will transport you to a world of richness and wonder. The spirulina in this eye shadow is the source of the beautiful aquamarine color in this recipe.

what you will need

- Six 3-ml glass cosmetic containers with lids
- Double boiler*
- Pipette
- ½ tsp avocado butter
- ½ tsp cocoa butter
- 1 tsp vegetable emulsifying wax
- ⅛ tsp magnesium stearate
- 1 tbsp (15 ml) aloe vera gel

- 10 drops rosehip oil
- 5 drops vitamin E oil
- 5 drops pomegranate oil
- ⅛ tsp arrowroot powder
- ¼ tsp mica powder (gold)
- ½ tsp mica powder (blue)
- ¼ tsp kaolin clay
- ½ tsp spirulina

MAKES SIX 3-ML COSMETIC CONTAINERS

step by step

1. In a double boiler over medium heat, completely melt the avocado butter, cocoa butter, and vegetable emulsifying wax.

2. Add the magnesium stearate while the mixture is still over the heat. Stir until completely incorporated. Remove from the heat.

3. While the mixture is still warm and melted, add the aloe vera gel, rosehip oil, vitamin E oil, and pomegranate oil. Stir until completely incorporated.

4. While the mixture is still warm and melted, add the arrowroot powder, mica powders, kaolin clay, and spirulina. Stir until completely incorporated.

5. Transfer the mixture to the cosmetic containers using a pipette and carefully add the lid.

6. Wait at least 60 minutes for the eye shadow to harden.

how to use Apply to clean, dry eyelids (or eyelids that have been prepped with eye shadow primer) using your finger. Blend well.

tip Try using this cream eye shadow as an eyeliner for green or brown eyes for a captivating impact.

modification Remove the mica powders for a bold swatch of green.

* See page 18 for instructions.

queen bee
powder eye shadow

You might think that you don't need a yellow eye shadow in your makeup repertoire, but have you ever tried one? The shade is softer than you might imagine and will remind you of a bright spring day when the flowers have just begun to bloom and honeybees abound. Pack a picnic because this eye shadow brings the sunshine.

what you will need

- Six 3-ml cosmetic containers with lids
- 1 tsp arrowroot powder
- ¼ tsp silica
- ¼ tsp turmeric
- ¼ tsp mica powder (yellow)

- ¼ tsp mica powder (gold)
- 5 drops rosehip oil
- 5 drops vitamin E oil
- 5 drops pomegranate oil

MAKES SIX 3-ML COSMETIC CONTAINERS

step by step

1. In a small mixing bowl, whisk together the arrowroot powder, silica, turmeric, and mica powders.

2. Add the rosehip oil, vitamin E oil, and pomegranate oil. Whisk together until fully incorporated.

3. Transfer the eye shadow to the cosmetic containers.

how to use Using an eye shadow brush (or your finger), apply shadow to lids.

tip Try pairing a yellow lid with a soft pink lip for a sweet springtime look. Apply the shadow with a damp liner brush along the upper lash line for a bold pop of color.

modification Remove the gold mica powder for a matte yellow shadow that pops. Increase the amount of yellow mica powder for a bolder yellow. Omit the turmeric if you want a cooler eye shadow instead of one with warmer undertones.

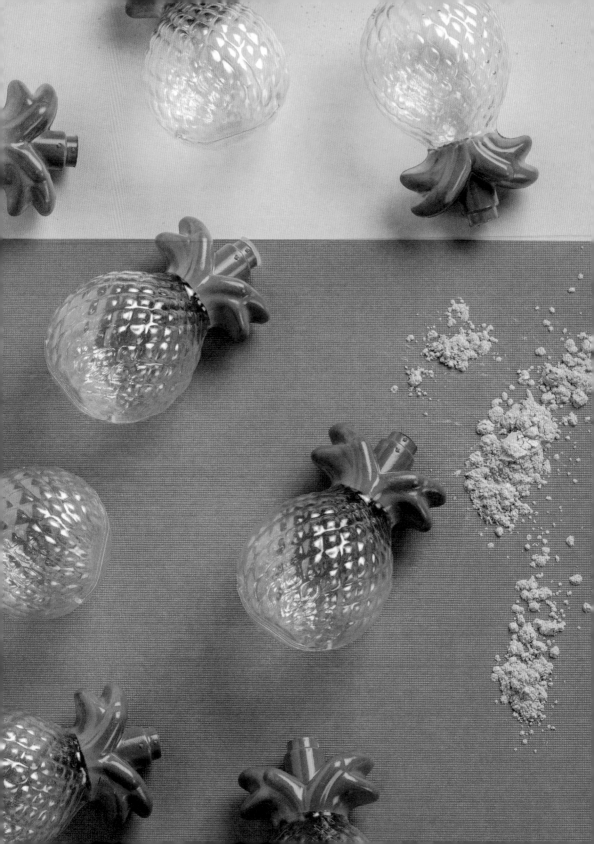

pineapple pop cream eye shadow

This eye shadow is sure to make you feel as if it's the middle of summer even if the skies are gray. This canary yellow cream shadow gets its bold base from turmeric and softening qualities from pomegranate oil and avocado butter.

what you will need

- Six 3-ml glass cosmetic containers with lids
- Double boiler*
- Pipette
- ½ tsp avocado butter
- ½ tsp cocoa butter
- 1 tsp vegetable emulsifying wax
- ⅛ tsp magnesium stearate

- 1 tbsp (15 ml) aloe vera gel
- 10 drops rosehip oil
- 5 drops vitamin E oil
- 5 drops pomegranate oil
- ⅛ tsp arrowroot powder
- ½ tsp mica powder (yellow)
- ½ tsp turmeric

MAKES SIX 3-ML COSMETIC CONTAINERS

step by step

1. In a double boiler over medium heat, completely melt the avocado butter, cocoa butter, and vegetable emulsifying wax.

2. Add the magnesium stearate while the mixture is still over the heat. Stir until completely incorporated. Remove from the heat.

3. While the mixture is still warm and melted, add the aloe vera gel, rosehip oil, vitamin E oil, and pomegranate oil. Stir until completely incorporated.

4. While the mixture is still warm and melted, add the arrowroot powder, mica powder, and turmeric. Stir until completely incorporated.

5. Transfer the mixture to the cosmetic containers using a pipette and carefully add the lid.

6. Wait at least 60 minutes for the eye shadow to harden.

how to use Apply to clean, dry eyelids (or eyelids that have been prepped with eye shadow primer) using your finger. Blend well.

tip Pair this peppy yellow with a bare face for an artistic statement. Use this yellow color on the tops of cheekbones for a unique blush and highlighter.

modification Try a contrasting shimmery mica powder—in hot pink or green—for a really wild cream eye shadow that is perfect for a playful party. Add iridescent mica powder for a shimmery look perfect for summer nights.

* See page 18 for instructions.

lilac macaron dream powder eye shadow

This pale purple is soft enough to be worn every day, but still makes a powerful pastel statement. Your lids will look like a watercolor painting awash in luminous lilac. Violet hues are beautiful on all eye colors, but this one really makes brown eyes pop.

what you will need

- Six 3-ml cosmetic containers with lids
- 1 tsp arrowroot powder
- ¼ tsp silica
- ½ tsp mica powder (purple matte)
- ¼ tsp mica powder (iridescent violet)
- 5 drops rosehip oil
- 5 drops vitamin E oil
- 5 drops pomegranate oil

MAKES SIX 3-ML COSMETIC CONTAINERS

EYE SHADOWS

step by step

1. In a small mixing bowl, whisk together the arrowroot powder, silica, and mica powders.

2. Add the rosehip oil, vitamin E oil, and pomegranate oil. Whisk together until fully incorporated.

3. Transfer the eye shadow to the cosmetic containers.

how to use Using an eye shadow brush (or your finger), apply shadow to lids.

tip If you have brown eyes, this eye shadow will make your eyes pop. This color is a universally flattering shade. Try lightly dusting it on the apples of the cheeks, as violet blush is surprisingly chic!

modification You can add a couple of drops of lavender oil to this shadow for a look that has a luscious scent to match. Double the amount of purple matte mica powder for a deeper purple, which looks great if you have dark brown eyes.

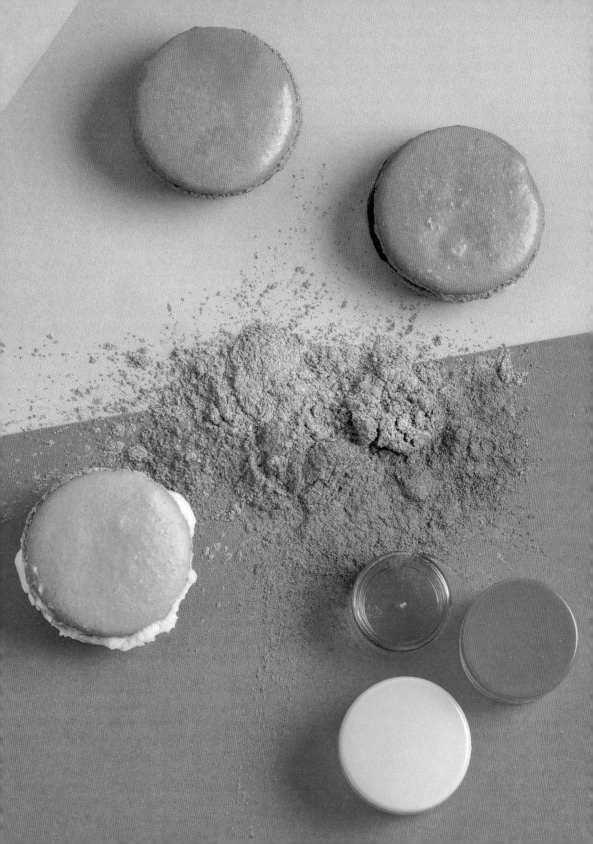

party from dusk 'til dawn cream eye shadow

This purple eye shadow feels a little rebellious. It's perfect for those days when you just need to let loose. And nothing says "let loose" like this sparkly purple shade.

what you will need

- Six 3-ml glass cosmetic containers with lids
- Double boiler*
- Pipette
- ½ tsp avocado butter
- ½ tsp cocoa butter
- 1 tsp vegetable emulsifying wax
- ⅛ tsp magnesium stearate
- 1 tbsp (15 ml) aloe vera gel
- 10 drops rosehip oil
- 5 drops vitamin E oil
- 5 drops pomegranate oil
- ⅛ tsp arrowroot powder
- ½ tsp mica powder (purple matte)
- ½ tsp mica powder (iridescent violet)

MAKES SIX 3-ML COSMETIC CONTAINERS

EYE SHADOWS

step by step

1. In a double boiler over medium heat, completely melt the avocado butter, cocoa butter, and vegetable emulsifying wax.

2. Add the magnesium stearate while the mixture is still over the heat. Stir until completely incorporated. Remove from the heat.

3. While the mixture is still warm and melted, add the aloe vera gel, rosehip oil, vitamin E oil, and pomegranate oil. Stir until completely incorporated.

4. While the mixture is still warm and melted, add the arrowroot powder and mica powders. Stir until completely incorporated.

5. Transfer the mixture to the cosmetic containers using a pipette and carefully add the lid.

6. Wait at least 60 minutes for the eye shadow to harden.

how to use Apply to clean, dry eyelids (or eyelids that have been prepped with eye shadow primer) using your finger. Blend well.

tip Pat this eye shadow onto your eyelids for a more intense effect. Use this shadow as a highlighter on the tippy-top of the cheekbone for a unicorn-like shine.

modification Add some blue and green mica powders to the recipe for a fun mix of colors—flashy like a peacock's feathers. Double the amount of iridescent violet mica powder for eyes that look like a glittering purple disco ball.

* See page 18 for instructions.

cocoa craze
cream eye shadow

Chocolate is one of the most delicious treats. When you have a chocolate craving, try reaching for this cocoa-colored (and -scented!) cream eye shadow. With a tiny hint of gold shimmer you might be so distracted that you forget you were craving chocolate in the first place!

what you will need

- Six 3-ml glass cosmetic containers with lids
- Double boiler*
- Pipette
- ½ tsp avocado butter
- ½ tsp cocoa butter
- 1 tsp vegetable emulsifying wax
- ⅛ tsp magnesium stearate
- 1 tbsp (15 ml) aloe vera gel

- 10 drops rosehip oil
- 5 drops vitamin E oil
- 5 drops pomegranate oil
- ⅛ tsp arrowroot powder
- ¼ tsp mica powder (gold)
- ¼ tsp kaolin clay
- ½ tsp cocoa powder

MAKES SIX 3-ML COSMETIC CONTAINERS

step by step

1. In a double boiler over medium heat, completely melt the avocado butter, cocoa butter, and vegetable emulsifying wax.

2. Add the magnesium stearate while the mixture is still over the heat. Stir until completely incorporated. Remove from the heat.

3. While the mixture is still warm and melted, add the aloe vera gel, rosehip oil, vitamin E oil, and pomegranate oil. Stir until completely incorporated.

4. While the mixture is still warm and melted, add the arrowroot powder, mica powder, kaolin clay, and cocoa powder. Stir until completely incorporated.

5. Transfer the mixture to the cosmetic containers using a pipette and carefully add the lid.

6. Wait at least 60 minutes for the eye shadow to harden.

how to use Apply to clean, dry eyelids (or eyelids that have been prepped with eye shadow primer) using your finger. Blend well.

tip This eye shadow can double as a shimmery contouring cream.

modification Double the amount of mica powder for a sparkly brown that might quickly become your go-to shade.

* See page 18 for instructions.

113

caramel crunch
powder eye shadow

If you're looking to add something sweet to your day, this eye shadow is the perfect solution. Soft browns swirl with majestic golds for an eye shadow neutral that is anything but. Apply liberally over the lid up to the brow bone for a captivating wash of color.

what you will need

- Six 3-ml cosmetic containers with lids
- 1 tsp arrowroot powder
- ¼ tsp silica
- ¼ tsp kaolin clay
- ½ tsp cocoa powder
- ¼ tsp mica powder (gold)
- 5 drops rosehip oil
- 5 drops vitamin E oil
- 5 drops pomegranate oil

MAKES SIX 3-ML COSMETIC CONTAINERS

step by step

1. In a small mixing bowl, whisk together the arrowroot powder, silica, kaolin clay, cocoa powder, and mica powder.

2. Add the rosehip oil, vitamin E oil, and pomegranate oil. Whisk together until fully incorporated.

3. Transfer the eye shadow to the cosmetic containers.

how to use Using an eye shadow brush (or your finger), apply shadow to lids.

tip This is your perfect everyday shadow. It has the right amount of shimmer and a soft brown tint. You can use a finger to rub it onto your upper lid and softly up to your brow line for a quick, polished look. This shadow is a beautiful all-over color that suits every skin shade. Use it on lips, lids, and cheeks for a quick makeup look.

modification Double the amount of mica powder and you have a bronze highlighter. Are you into all things matte? Simply remove the mica powder.

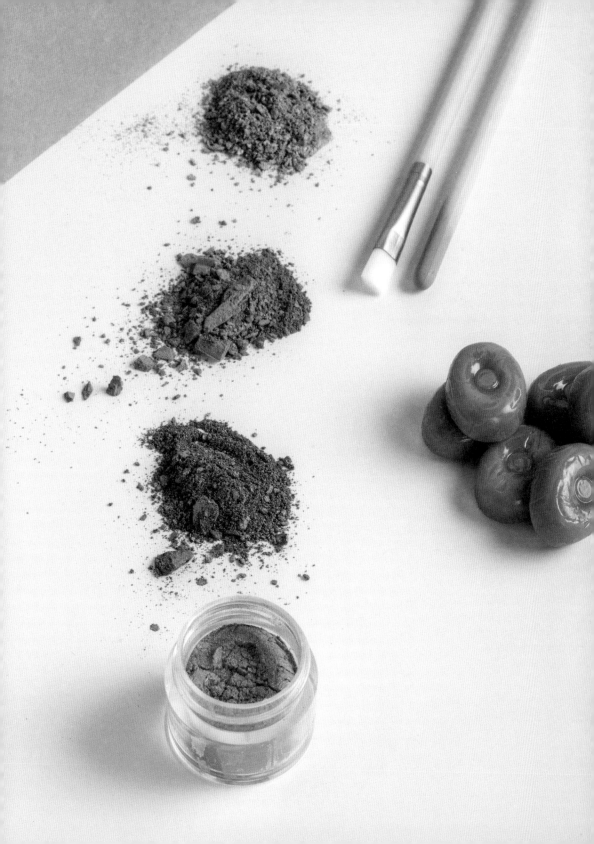

flamingo floatie cream eye shadow

The deep pink in this little pot of color will remind you of the Instagram-worthy flamingo floaties snapped at a pool party. Even if your life doesn't include a daily plunge into chlorine-filled bliss, you can still channel some festive vibes with this bold, pink hue.

what you will need

- Six 3-ml glass cosmetic containers with lids
- Double boiler*
- Pipette
- ½ tsp avocado butter
- ½ tsp cocoa butter
- 1 tsp vegetable emulsifying wax
- ⅛ tsp magnesium stearate
- 1 tbsp (15 ml) aloe vera gel
- 10 drops rosehip oil
- 5 drops vitamin E oil
- 5 drops pomegranate oil
- ⅛ tsp arrowroot powder
- ½ tsp mica powder (pink)
- ½ tsp beetroot powder

MAKES SIX 3-ML COSMETIC CONTAINERS

step by step

1. In a double boiler over medium heat, completely melt the avocado butter, cocoa butter, and vegetable emulsifying wax.

2. Add the magnesium stearate while the mixture is still over the heat. Stir until completely incorporated. Remove from the heat.

3. While the mixture is still warm and melted, add the aloe vera gel, rosehip oil, vitamin E oil, and pomegranate oil. Stir until completely incorporated.

4. While the mixture is still warm and melted, add the arrowroot powder, mica powder, and beetroot powder. Stir until completely incorporated.

5. Transfer the mixture to the cosmetic containers using a pipette and carefully add the lid.

6. Wait at least 60 minutes for the eye shadow to harden.

how to use Apply to clean, dry eyelids (or eyelids that have been prepped with eye shadow primer) using your finger. Blend well.

tip Pat this on the center of your eyelid and blend slightly outward to the corners of your eye for an ombré effect.

modification Add iridescent mica powder to this recipe for a super-girly pink.

* See page 18 for instructions.

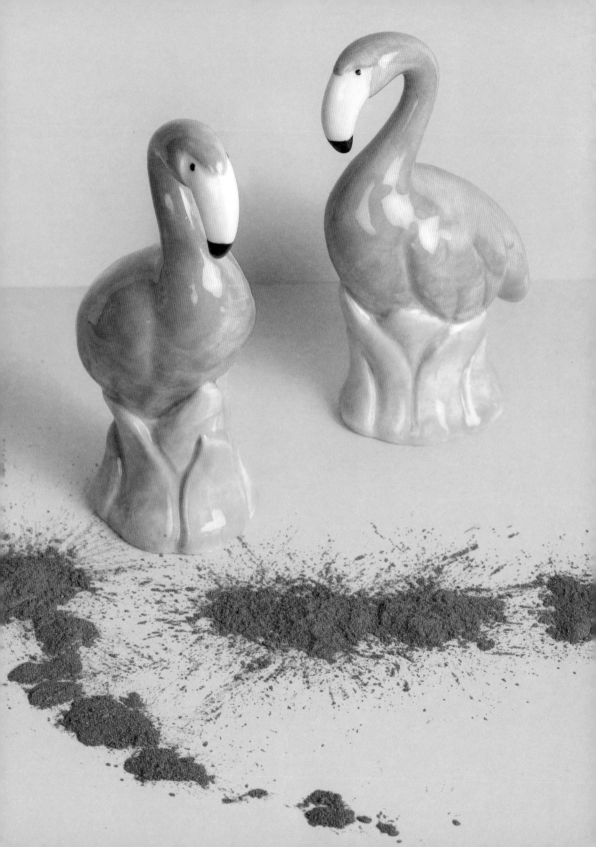

pink perfection
powder eye shadow

Forty years ago, hot pink had its moment. (Or, more accurately, it's decade.) The '80s were full of this bright tone, and it's time to bring it back. To keep this look modern, pair this loud pink with a neutral lip and a light dusting of bronzer for a look that is decidedly now. Fun fact: we have an '80s playlist that we listen to on our way to school!

what you will need

- Six 3-ml cosmetic containers with lids
- 1 tsp arrowroot powder
- ¼ tsp silica
- ¼ tsp kaolin clay
- ½ tsp beetroot powder

- ¼ tsp mica powder (pink)
- 5 drops rosehip oil
- 5 drops vitamin E oil
- 5 drops pomegranate oil

MAKES SIX 3-ML COSMETIC CONTAINERS

step by step

1. In a small mixing bowl, whisk together the arrowroot powder, silica, kaolin clay, beetroot powder, and mica powder.

2. Add the rosehip oil, vitamin E oil, and pomegranate oil. Whisk together until fully incorporated.

3. Transfer the eye shadow to the cosmetic containers.

how to use Using an eye shadow brush (or your finger), apply shadow to lids.

tip For an unexpected look, cover lids with a neutral eye shadow and use this hot-pink eye shadow on the inner corners of your eyes. This strategic placement of color makes for a modern look.

modification To use this shadow as a matte rouge, remove the mica powder. It works beautifully on cheeks!

shimmer n' shine 24k cream eye shadow

It can be fun to play with your look, but the key to true beauty is a heart of gold. Wear your heart on your sleeve (or your lids!) with this super sparkly cream eye shadow.

what you will need

- Six 3-ml glass cosmetic containers with lids
- Double boiler*
- Pipette
- ½ tsp avocado butter
- ½ tsp cocoa butter
- 1 tsp vegetable emulsifying wax
- ⅛ tsp magnesium stearate

- 1 tbsp (15 ml) aloe vera gel
- 10 drops rosehip oil
- 5 drops vitamin E oil
- 5 drops pomegranate oil
- ⅛ tsp arrowroot powder
- 1 tsp mica powder (gold)

MAKES SIX 3-ML COSMETIC CONTAINERS

step by step

1. In a double boiler over medium heat, completely melt the avocado butter, cocoa butter, and vegetable emulsifying wax.

2. Add the magnesium stearate while the mixture is still over the heat. Stir until completely incorporated. Remove from the heat.

3. While the mixture is still warm and melted, add the aloe vera gel, rosehip oil, vitamin E oil, and pomegranate oil. Stir until completely incorporated.

4. While the mixture is still warm and melted, add the arrowroot powder and mica powder. Stir until completely incorporated.

5. Transfer the mixture to the cosmetic containers using a pipette and carefully add the lid.

6. Wait at least 60 minutes for the eye shadow to harden.

how to use Apply to clean, dry eyelids (or eyelids that have been prepped with eye shadow primer) using your finger. Blend well.

tip Try layering this creamy shimmer over other shades for a multidimensional look.

modification Want even more sparkle? Add more gold mica powder until you reach your desired level of shine.

* See page 18 for instructions.

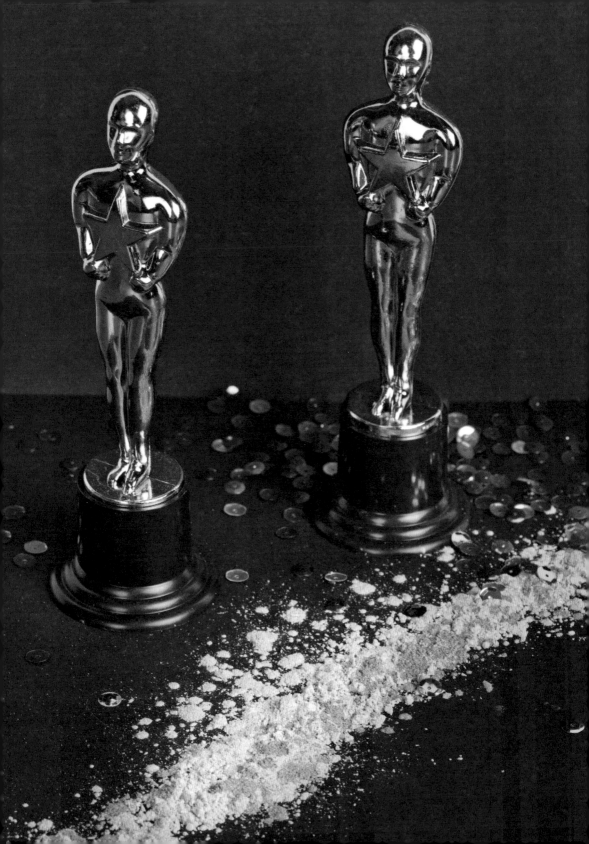

and the oscar goes to . . . powder eye shadow

There's no doubt you'll win the glam award when you slide on this shimmery gold shadow. It looks gorgeous alone or layered over other colors. Try applying this shadow all the way from your lid to your brow bone for a red carpet-worthy look.

what you will need

- Six 3-ml cosmetic containers with lids
- 1 tsp arrowroot powder
- ¼ tsp silica
- ½ tsp mica powder (gold)

- 5 drops rosehip oil
- 5 drops vitamin E oil
- 5 drops pomegranate oil

MAKES SIX 3-ML COSMETIC CONTAINERS

step by step

1. In a small mixing bowl, whisk together the arrowroot powder, silica, and mica powder.

2. Add the rosehip oil, vitamin E oil, and pomegranate oil. Whisk together until fully incorporated.

3. Transfer the eye shadow to the cosmetic containers.

how to use Using an eye shadow brush (or your finger), apply shadow to lids.

tip You can also use this as a highlighter or dust it across the shoulders and chest with a large fluffy brush for subtle skin shimmer.

modification The amount of sparkle is up to you. If you like things a little more subtle, decrease the amount of mica powder. Like a lot of shimmer? Double the amount of mica powder!

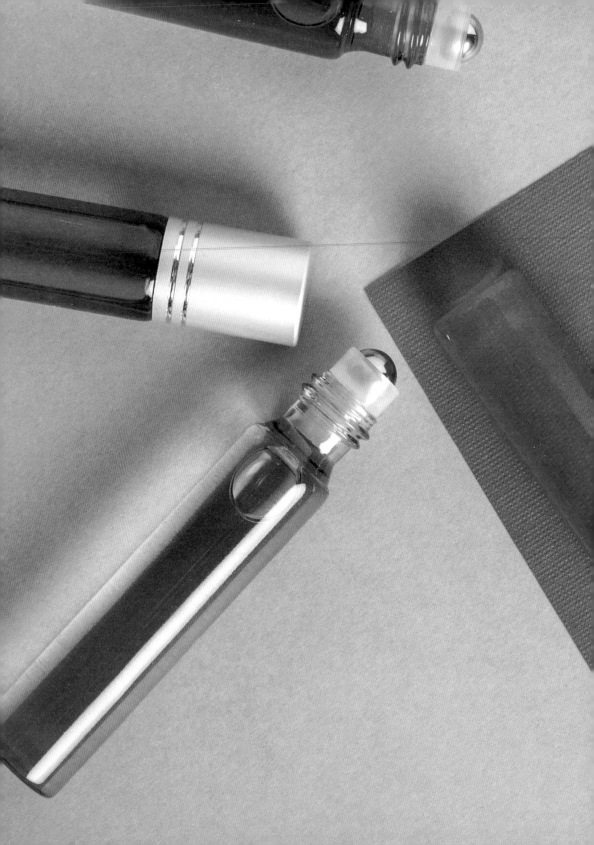

SKIN CARE

Caroline's personal favorite, skin care is the baseline to keeping your skin healthy and prepped for a smooth makeup look. It's always fun to be able to customize your skin care routine to suit your complexion. (And your skin will thank you!)

i woke up like this face mask

Brighten up your skin with this mask full of natural exfoliants like papaya and lemon. These super fruits help with skin cell turnover, the avocado and honey provide moisture, and the cinnamon fights bacteria.

what you will need

- Blender
- ¼ papaya
- 2 tsp honey
- ½ avocado
- ½ tsp turmeric
- 1 tsp lemon juice
- ½ tsp ground cinnamon

MAKES ONE MASK

step by step

1. Put all the ingredients into a blender.
2. Blend to create a smooth paste.

how to use Put the mask on clean, dry skin. Leave on for 10 to 15 minutes. Rinse off with warm water and a washcloth.

tip You can rub this mask into your skin before allowing it to set. This allows the ingredients to act as natural exfoliants.

modification If you can't find a papaya in your neck of the woods, double the amount of avocado.

so fresh, so clean face mask

This mask uses three simple ingredients to deeply clean the face. All three ingredients—coconut oil, lemon juice, and raw honey—have natural antibacterial properties. What does this mean for your skin? It means that this simple mask is incredible at getting rid of dirt, toxins, and acne-causing bacteria. Your face will feel brand new after you indulge in some self-care with this mask.

what you will need

- 2 tsp coconut oil
- ½ tsp lemon juice
- ½ tsp raw honey

MAKES ONE MASK

step by step

1. Put all the ingredients into a mixing bowl.
2. Mix well until incorporated.

how to use Gently massage into clean, dry skin. Leave on for up to 30 minutes. Rinse with warm water and a clean washcloth.

tip Try using this mask twice a week for a month. You'll likely notice a difference—less acne and a smoother, more even complexion.

modification Add a few drops of lavender essential oil for an antibacterial boost.

moisture, please! face mask

This mask—made with ingredients you can find in your kitchen—proves that eating healthy food isn't the only way to extract powerful beauty benefits. Each ingredient in this recipe is known for its hydrating properties. When you combine all four of these and let them soak in, the result is wonderfully plumped, hydrated skin.

what you will need

- ½ banana
- ¼ avocado
- 1 tsp honey
- 1 tsp aloe vera gel

MAKES ONE MASK

step by step

1. Put all the ingredients in a mixing bowl.
2. Mash with a fork until fully incorporated.

how to use Lie down with a towel under your head. This mask is not a fan of gravity and can get a little bit messy. Massage the mask onto your skin and keep your head still. Leave on for 5 to 10 minutes. Rinse with warm water and pat dry with a washcloth.

tip Use this mask once a week during dry winter months to combat dehydrating weather.

modification If avocado is hard to find, double the amount of banana or try mixing in plain yogurt.

forever young face mask

If you really want to get ahead of the aging game, set aside 10 minutes a week for some self-care and relaxation time—with this mask on your face. Avocado and yogurt hydrate, lemon fights discoloration, honey destroys bacteria, and witch hazel shrinks pores. This super powerful light-green mask will keep you feeling (and looking!) forever young.

what you will need

- ¼ avocado
- 1 tsp honey
- ½ tsp lemon juice
- ¼ cup (60 g) plain yogurt
- ½ tsp witch hazel

MAKES ONE MASK

step by step

1. Put all the ingredients into a mixing bowl.
2. Mix well until incorporated.

how to use Place a thin layer of the mask on clean, dry skin. Leave on your face and neck for 10 minutes. Rinse with warm water and pat dry with a washcloth.

tip Want to really help this mask sink into the skin? Place a warm washcloth over your face for 2 minutes to open your pores before applying this face mask.

modification You can leave out the avocado if it isn't in season or available near you. Add 1 tbsp (15 g) of yogurt instead.

sherbet swirl face mask

Some days you just need to kick back, unwind, and let a face mask do all the work. For those days when your life and your skin need something extra soothing, try this calming mask. It smells good enough to eat—since all the ingredients are edible!

what you will need

- Blender
- 1 tsp honey
- 2 tsp cocoa powder
- ¼ banana
- ¼ peeled cucumber
- ¼ cup (60 g) plain yogurt

MAKES ONE MASK

step by step

1. Place all the ingredients in a blender.
2. Blend briefly. Stop the blender when the ingredients have formed a thick paste.

how to use Put the mask on clean, dry skin. Leave on as long as you like—a minimum of 5 minutes is recommended. Rinse well with warm water and pat dry with a clean washcloth. Follow with toner and moisturizer.

tip This mask can get messy! Make sure you lie down with your hair tied back and a towel under your head to catch any drips.

modification You can put this mask in the fridge for an hour for an extra-chilly soothing sensation.

pore be gone face mask

If you're on a mission to shrink your pores—which can easily grow larger with cosmetic use, dirt, or environmental pollution—then this mask is exactly what you need. All of the ingredients in this deep-cleaning addition to your skin care routine help clear the pores and keep them clean. With regular use, you may need a magnifying glass to find your pores.

what you will need

- 1 tsp activated charcoal
- 1 tsp zinc oxide
- 1 tsp kaolin clay
- 2 tsp witch hazel

MAKES ONE MASK

step by step

1. Put all the ingredients in a mixing bowl.
2. Mix well until fully incorporated.

how to use Put the mask on clean, dry skin, focusing on areas that are prone to blackheads. For most people this area is the T-zone (nose and area between the eyebrows), the sides of the nose near the cheeks, and the chin.

tip Try using this mask after you have exfoliated your skin for an even deeper clean.

modification Add a couple of drops of lavender oil and tea tree oil to help kill bacteria and shrink pores.

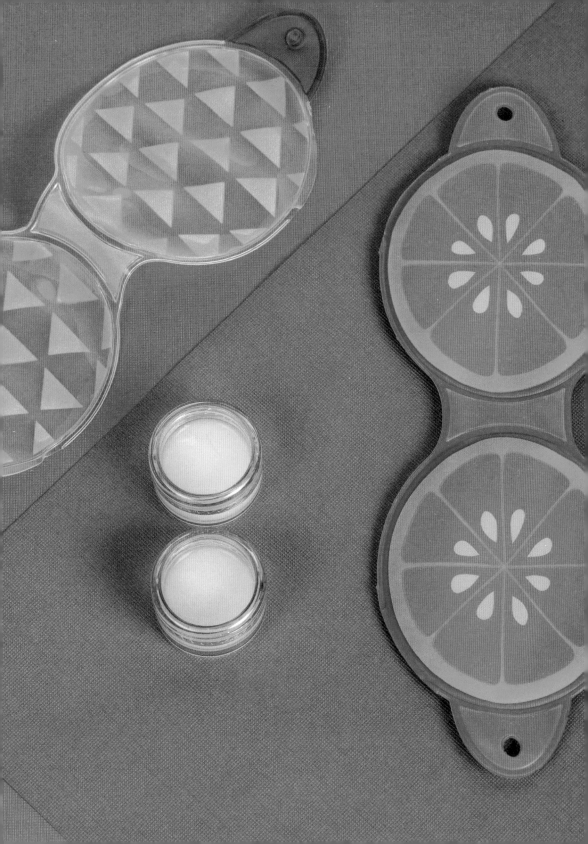

sacred skin daily serum

This serum can be your secret to absolutely radiant skin. The oils in this blend have antiaging, antibacterial, and antioxidant benefits.

what you will need

- 4-oz (120-ml) bottle with dropper lid
- Dropper
- 1 tbsp (15 ml) olive oil
- 1 tbsp (15 ml) lavender oil
- 1 tbsp (15 ml) rosemary oil
- 2 tbsp (30 ml) jojoba oil
- 2 tbsp (30 ml) avocado oil
- 1 tbsp (15 ml) raspberry seed oil

MAKES ONE 4-OUNCE (120-ML) CONTAINER

step by step

1. Use the dropper to transfer the oils to the bottle.

2. Put the lid on the bottle and shake well to incorporate the oils.

how to use Place 5 to 10 drops in your palms and warm the serum. Press into clean, dry skin.

tip For the best results, apply serum after your morning skin-care routine, which should involve cleansing and toning.

modification Have a favorite oil for your skin? Feel free to add it in! You can mix and match the oils in the serum until you have the perfect combination.

sleeping beauty serum

A full night of sleep with this serum soaking into your skin will have you waking up looking like you got all the beauty sleep you could ever need.

what you will need

- 4-oz (120-ml) bottle with dropper lid
- Dropper
- 4 tbsp (60 ml) rosehip oil
- 4 tbsp (60 ml) argan oil
- 30 drops lavender oil

MAKES ONE 4-OUNCE (120-ML) CONTAINER

step by step

1. Use the dropper to transfer the oils to the bottle.

2. Put the lid on the bottle and shake well to incorporate the oils.

how to use Place 5 to 10 drops in your palms and warm the serum. Press into clean, dry skin.

tip For the best results, apply serum after your evening skin-care routine, which should involve cleansing and toning.

modification Want extra overnight skin benefits? Spring for some frankincense oil and add some to this mix. It is skin magic.

hydrated hunny serum

Quench your skin's thirst with this ultra-moisturizing face serum.

what you will need

- 4-oz (120-ml) bottle with dropper lid
- Dropper
- 2 tbsp (30 ml) rosehip oil
- 2 tbsp (30 ml) almond oil
- 1 tbsp (15 ml) avocado oil
- 2 tsp carrot seed oil
- 1 tsp jasmine oil
- 2 tbsp (30 ml) kukui oil

MAKES ONE 4-OUNCE (120-ML) CONTAINER

step by step

1. Use the dropper to transfer the oils to the bottle.

2. Put the lid on the bottle and shake well to incorporate the oils.

how to use Place 5 to 10 drops in your palms and warm the serum. Press into clean, dry skin.

tip This luxurious oil can also be used on the neck and chest for some serious hydration.

modification Jasmine isn't your scent of choice? Try different skin-safe essential oils until a fragrance suits your senses.

so bright, so tight serum

This serum makes you look lit from within. Lemon oil brightens while argan oil and vitamin E oil hydrate and stop aging in its tracks.

what you will need

- 4-oz (120-ml) bottle with dropper lid
- Dropper
- 7 tbsp (105 ml) argan oil
- 2 tsp lemon oil
- 1 tsp vitamin E oil

MAKES ONE 4-OUNCE (120-ML) CONTAINER

step by step

1. Use the dropper to transfer the oils and the vitamin E oil to the bottle.

2. Put the lid on the bottle and shake well to incorporate the oils.

how to use Place 5 to 10 drops in your palms and warm the serum. Press into clean, dry skin.

tip This oil helps even your skin tone and brighten any areas of discoloration. For the most impact, apply this serum at night to let the lemon oil work its skin-brightening magic.

modification You can add a few drops of pomelo oil for a light scent that also helps brighten skin.

bye, bye bumps serum

The right oils can help balance your skin's natural oil production and, in turn, help stop acne in its tracks.

what you will need

- 4-oz (120-ml) bottle with dropper lid
- Dropper
- 2 tbsp (30 ml) rosehip oil
- 2 tbsp (30 ml) kukui oil
- 1 tbsp (15 ml) rosemary oil
- 2 tbsp (30 ml) carrot seed oil
- 1 tsp eucalyptus oil
- 2 tsp jasmine oil

MAKES ONE 4-OUNCE (120-ML) CONTAINER

step by step

1. Use the dropper to transfer the oils to the bottle.

2. Put the lid on the bottle and shake well to incorporate the oils.

how to use Place 5 to 10 drops in your palms and warm the serum. Press into clean, dry skin.

tip This oil is strong on acne but gentle enough to be used every day.

modification You can add a few drops of tea tree oil for added acne-blasting benefits.

no problem exfoliant

Keep your skin looking fresh with this gentle exfoliant. The sugar is a natural exfoliator and the lemon oil is antibacterial and brightening!

what you will need

- 8-oz (240-ml) jar with lid
- 10 tbsp (150 ml) coconut oil
- 6 tbsp (75 g) cane sugar
- 2 tsp lemon oil

MAKES ONE 8-OUNCE (240-ML) JAR

how to use After cleansing skin, rub 1 tbsp (15 g) of the exfoliant on your face and neck in circular motions. Avoid the eyes. After rubbing thoroughly, rinse well with warm water and pat dry. Follow with a toner.

tip This exfoliant is gentle enough to use up to three times a week.

modification Add a few drops of eucalyptus oil for an exfoliant that is also a quick sensory wake-up.

step by step

1. Place all the ingredients in a jar.

2. Stir well to incorporate the ingredients.

new skin, new me exfoliant

In this exfoliant, coffee and cane sugar help slough off dead skin cells, honey keeps bacteria in check, and olive oil hydrates and fights fine lines.

what you will need

- 8-oz (240-ml) jar with lid
- 3 tbsp (45 ml) olive oil
- 5 tbsp (60 g) cane sugar
- 2 tsp honey
- ¼ cup (30 g) ground coffee

MAKES ONE 8-OUNCE (240-ML) JAR

step by step

1. Place all the ingredients in a jar.
2. Stir well to incorporate the ingredients.

how to use After cleansing your skin, rub 1 tbsp (15 g) of the exfoliant on your face and neck in circular motions. Avoid the eyes. After rubbing thoroughly, rinse well with warm water and pat dry. Follow with a toner.

miss me, kiss me lip scrub

In a standard skin care routine, the mouth often gets overlooked. Lips can show signs of fatigue and aging, so their sensitive skin should get some extra attention.

what you will need

- 50-gram container with lid
- 2 tbsp (25 g) raw sugar
- 2 tsp honey
- 1 tbsp (15 ml) olive oil

MAKES ONE 50-GRAM CONTAINER

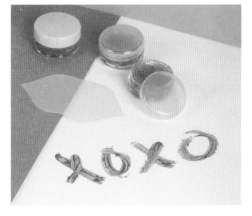

step by step

1. Place all the ingredients in a container.
2. Stir well until fully incorporated.

how to use Take a small amount of the mixture and apply to clean, dry lips. Gently rub all over lips in a circular motion. Rinse off using a warm washcloth.

tip Immediately after exfoliating the lips, apply a hydrating balm to lock in the effect.

modification Add a few drops of vitamin E oil to hydrate and soften the lips as you smooth them.

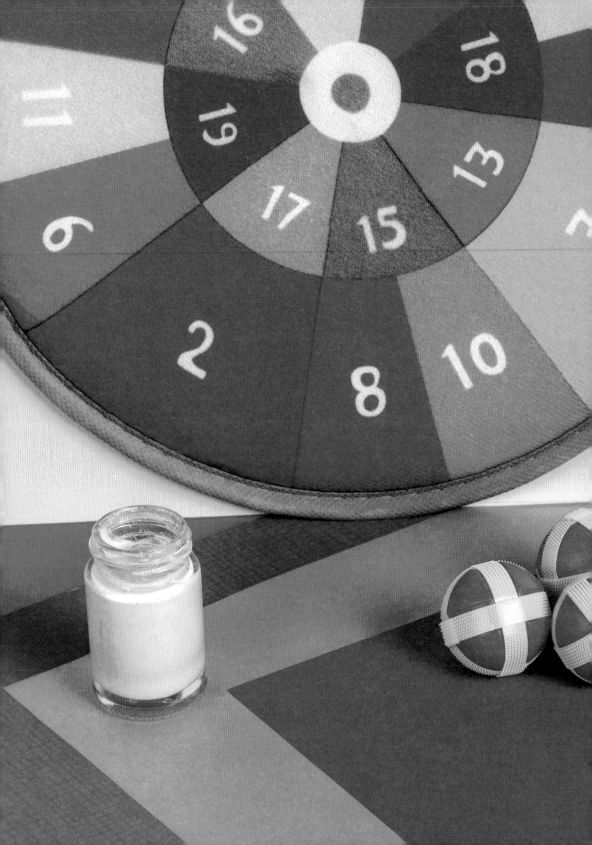

eyes on the prize
spot treatment

This amazing acne-crushing spot treatment can work overnight. It doesn't leave anything to chance—it dries up the oil that contributes to blemishes, kills the bacteria, hydrates the skin, and reduces redness.

what you will need

- 4-oz (120-ml) bottle with dropper lid
- Dropper
- 1 tbsp (15 ml) tea tree oil
- 7 tbsp (105 ml) calamine lotion

MAKES ONE 4-OUNCE (120-ML) BOTTLE

step by step

1. Put the tea tree oil and calamine lotion in a mixing bowl.

2. Mix well until the ingredients are fully incorporated.

3. Using a dropper, transfer the mixture to the bottle.

how to use After cleansing and toning your skin at night, use the dropper to put this mixture on a cotton swab. Press the cotton swab gently against any spots or blemishes and allow time to dry before going to bed. Rinse off with warm water upon waking.

tip Feel a blemish brewing beneath the surface? This treatment can dry out a blemish and get rid of the bacteria before it appears! Apply at night after cleansing and toning to any areas of the face that are acne prone (to get ahead of any blemishes that may be brewing!).

modification You can add a few drops of lavender oil for bacteria-fighting benefits and a soothing aroma that will help lull you to sleep. A few drops of lemon oil can pack a double punch. The antibacterial element busts acne-causing bacteria and also helps lighten any scarring.

bye dry skin
soother treatment

This overnight treatment helps treat red spots and scarring on sensitive facial skin. The baking soda is healing and the oils work in combination with the aloe vera to soothe and restore.

what you will need

- 4-oz (120-ml) bottle with dropper lid
- Dropper
- 4 tbsp (60 ml) aloe vera gel
- 2 tsp baking soda
- 2 tbsp (30 ml) fractionated coconut oil
- 2 tbsp (30 ml) rosehip oil

MAKES ONE 4-OUNCE (120-ML) BOTTLE

step by step

1. Put the ingredients in a mixing bowl.

2. Mix well until fully incorporated.

3. Using a dropper, transfer the mixture to the bottle. Discard excess.

how to use After cleansing and toning at night, use the dropper to put this mixture on a cotton swab. Press the cotton swab gently against any red spots or scars and allow time to dry before going to bed. Rinse off with warm water upon waking.

tip You can use this spot treatment as a face mask for reducing redness. Put it on clean, dry skin and leave on for 10 minutes before rinsing off with warm water.

modification You can add ¼ tsp of vitamin E oil to help soothe acne scars.

bye, bye aging signs treatment

This hydrating balm harnesses the power of argan oil and vitamin E oil to fight dryness, fine lines, discoloration, and the signs of aging.

what you will need

- 50-gram glass cosmetic container with lid
- Double boiler*
- Funnel
- 1 tbsp (15 g) shea butter
- 1 tbsp (15 ml) coconut oil
- 1 tbsp (15 ml) aloe vera gel
- ¼ tsp argan oil
- ¼ tsp vitamin E oil

MAKES ONE 50-GRAM CONTAINER

See page 18 for instructions.

step by step

1. In a double boiler over medium heat, melt the shea butter and coconut oil until fully dissolved. Remove from the heat.

2. Stir in the aloe vera gel, argan oil, and vitamin E oil until fully incorporated.

3. Using a funnel, transfer the mixture to the cosmetic container and carefully add the lid.

4. Place immediately in the freezer for 30 minutes to harden the mixture.

how to use After cleansing and toning your skin, apply this balm to the area under the eyes.

bright eyes
undereye treatment

You already know that coffee is a quick way to get your day started or to perk yourself up after a long night. Did you know that the same caffeine that helps wake up your mind can also perk up your skin? Keep strongly brewed coffee frozen for the fastest way to get rid of bags and circles under your eyes.

what you will need

- Coffee maker
- Coffee
- Ice cube tray

MAKES ONE ICE CUBE TRAY OF COFFEE CUBES

step by step

1. Brew a pot of extra-strong coffee (twice the usual amount of ground coffee or beans).

2. Allow the coffee to cool to room temperature.

3. Pour the coffee into the ice cube tray.

4. Place the tray in the freezer.

5. You can use the cubes once they are completely frozen.

how to use Upon waking, hold an ice cube to the area under your eye for a few minutes or until the ice cube is melted. Repeat under the other eye.

tip You should do this over a bowl or the sink as the coffee ice cube melts. Had a long night? Do this treatment twice for extra cooling, caffeine-boosting benefits.

modification You can brew the coffee even stronger for a faster effect. You can use any coffee you like. Aroma is important, so try different blends and brews to find your favorite scent.

self-care salve

It is so important to take time for self-care. Part of this time should be spent caring for overlooked areas that may not normally make their way into your beauty routine. A lot of people forget to care for the delicate skin on the neck and chest. These areas need to be cared for because they can be the first areas to show signs of aging— and the neck and chest tend to absorb a lot of damaging UV rays. This luxurious salve is so hydrating, with such a creamy texture, you'll want to use it all the time.

what you will need

- 50-gram glass cosmetic container with lid
- Double boiler*
- 1 tsp shea butter
- 2 tsp vegetable emulsifying wax
- 2 tbsp (30 ml) coconut oil
- ¼ tsp silica
- ½ tsp argan oil

- ½ tsp jojoba oil
- ½ tsp sweet almond oil
- ½ tsp rosehip oil
- ½ tsp witch hazel
- 2 cups (480 ml) distilled water
- 1 tbsp (15 ml) aloe vera gel (clear)

MAKES ONE 50-GRAM CONTAINER

step by step

1. In a double boiler over medium heat, melt the shea butter, vegetable emulsifying wax, and coconut oil until fully dissolved. Remove from the heat.

2. Add the remaining ingredients and stir until fully incorporated.

3. Using a funnel, transfer the mixture to the cosmetic container and carefully add the lid.

4. Place immediately in the freezer for 30 minutes to harden the mixture.

how to use Apply to clean, dry skin on the neck and chest. Reapply as desired.

tip Apply this before bed so that it has time to soak in.

modification The neck and chest are commonly areas where perfume is placed. Add some of your favorite essential oils to this salve for a product that treats delicate skin and doubles as a perfume.

* See page 18 for instructions.

au naturel woman lash and brow growth treatment

Lashes and brows are having a huge beauty moment. If you aren't naturally blessed with long lashes and bushy brows, this treatment will get you where you want to be. Already blessed with the perfect eye fringe? This treatment conditions already existing hair and helps it stay hydrated and strong.

what you will need

- 10-ml mascara container with eyelash/eyebrow wand
- Small funnel or pipette
- 1 tsp castor oil
- ¾ tsp fractionated coconut oil
- ½ tsp vitamin E oil

MAKES ONE 10-ML CONTAINER

step by step

1. Place all the ingredients in a mixing bowl.

2. Stir until all the ingredients become liquid and incorporated.

3. Use a funnel or pipette to transfer the mixture to the mascara container.

how to use Apply to clean, dry lashes and brows at night before bed.

tropical hunny facial cleanser

Three simple ingredients—castile soap, coconut water, and honey—come together and work their magic to soften your skin. The castile soap foams and leaves you feeling squeaky clean.

what you will need

- 250-ml foam dispenser
- 3 tbsp (45 ml) castile soap
- ¾ cup (180 ml) coconut water
- ¼ tsp honey

MAKES ONE 250-ML DISPENSER

step by step

1. Put all the ingredients in the foam dispenser and gently tip back and forth to incorporate.

how to use Wet your face and pump the mixture into your hands. Rub all over your face and neck, forming a lather. Rinse well with warm water. You can use this cleanser alone or after oil cleansing.

tip Do not shake this mixture or the castile soap will turn to foam inside the dispenser.

modification Add ¼ tsp of vitamin E oil to this cleanser for extra hydration.

clean slate facial cleanser

We all deserve a second chance—and so does your skin. Lemon and honey are the two ingredients that get your skin back to square one. The lemon brightens and balances pH levels while the honey hydrates and battles acne and scarring.

what you will need

- 250-ml foam dispenser
- 3 tbsp (45 ml) castile soap
- ¾ cup (180 ml) distilled water
- ¼ tsp honey
- ¼ tsp lemon juice

MAKES ONE 250-ML DISPENSER

step by step

1. Put all the ingredients in the foam dispenser and gently tip back and forth to incorporate.

how to use Wet your face and pump the mixture into your hands. Rub all over your face and neck, forming a lather. Rinse well with warm water. You can use this cleanser alone or after oil cleansing.

tip Use this mixture within 10 days to avoid bacteria. Whip up a new batch when you're ready.

modification Add a few drops of lavender oil to the cleanser to stave off bacteria growth.

slick stuff oil cleanser

Have you ever tried oil cleansing? It's an ancient technique that removes dirt, makeup, and toxins while gently exfoliating and hydrating the skin. While you rub in the cleanser you are also performing facial massage, which helps bring healing blood flow to the skin's surface and reduces puffiness and inflammation in the face.

what you will need

- 8-oz (240 ml) jar with lid
- 2 tbsp (30 ml) castor oil
- 2 tbsp (30 ml) olive oil
- 2 tbsp (30 ml) jojoba oil
- 10 tbsp (150 ml) coconut oil

MAKES ONE 8-OUNCE (240 ML) JAR

step by step

1. Put all the ingredients into the jar.
2. Stir well until fully incorporated.

how to use Take 1 tbsp (15 ml) of the cleanser and rub into dry skin. Continue rubbing in a circular motion to dissolve dirt and makeup. Leave on skin for 1 to 3 minutes. Rinse with warm water. Pat dry with a washcloth.

tip It is normal to feel a remaining residue of oil on your skin. You can rub this in or allow it to sink in throughout the day. If you don't like how that feels, follow oil cleansing with a traditional cleanser to remove the oil.

modification You can add ¼ tsp of vitamin E oil for an oil cleanser with antiaging benefits.

facial in a jar cleansing balm

This balm does it all in one step. As it cleanses, it also exfoliates and hydrates. The coconut oil and beeswax pellets form the hydrating base of this balm. They also act as cleansing agents and destroy bacteria. The bentonite clay exfoliates and draws toxins out from deep beneath the skin's surface, helping reduce the size and appearance of pores. The jojoba oil and frankincense oil help lock in moisture, fight aging, and promote even skin tone.

what you will need

- 8-oz (240-ml) glass jar with lid
- 9 tbsp (135 ml) coconut oil
- 1 tbsp (15 g) beeswax pellets

- 2 tbsp (16 g) bentonite clay
- 2 tbsp (30 ml) jojoba oil
- 1 tsp frankincense oil

MAKES ONE 8-OUNCE (240-ML) JAR

step by step

1. Put the coconut oil and beeswax pellets into the glass jar.

2. Place the glass jar in a pot of hot water that comes halfway up the sides of the jar. Allow this water to fully melt the coconut oil and beeswax.

3. Remove the glass jar from the water and place on a heatproof surface.

4. Add the bentonite clay, jojoba oil, and frankincense oil. Stir until completely incorporated. Keep stirring slowly until the glass jar becomes cool enough to hold.

5. Carefully add the lid and transfer the glass jar to the freezer for 30 minutes to harden.

how to use Take 1 tbsp (15 g) of the cleansing balm and rub onto dry skin. Continue rubbing in a circular motion to dissolve dirt and makeup. Leave on skin for 1 to 3 minutes. Rinse with warm water. Pat dry with a washcloth.

tip It is normal to feel a remaining residue of oil on your skin. Rub this oil deeply into skin deeply.

modification Add a few drops of tea tree oil for a tingling cleansing experience.

so zen toner for normal skin

Keep your skin so balanced, people will think you've been meditating. The rose water in this simple toner helps keep your pH in check. The frankincense oil is thought to have antiaging properties. A few spritzes of this balanced mist will get your skin into a Zen state.

what you will need

- 4-oz (120-ml) bottle with spray top
- Funnel
- 7 tbsp (105 ml) rose water
- 1 tbsp (15 ml) frankincense oil

MAKES ONE 4-OUNCE (120-ML) BOTTLE

step by step

1. Using the funnel, transfer the rose water and frankincense oil to the bottle.

2. Shake well.

how to use Shake before use. Using the spray bottle or a cotton ball, apply toner all over freshly cleansed face and neck.

tip This toner can be used morning and night.

shine control toner

If your skin is on the oily side, it takes only a little bit of this liquid to get that oil in check. Apple cider vinegar and witch hazel work to combat oil production and shrink pores. If you use this mist daily, you might find that your skin has all the hydration it needs and begins to produce less oil. Who knew your skin was so smart?

what you will need

- 4-oz (120-ml) bottle with spray top
- Funnel
- 1 tsp apple cider vinegar
- 2 tbsp (30 ml) witch hazel
- 6 tbsp (90 ml) distilled water

MAKES ONE 4-OUNCE (120-ML) BOTTLE

step by step

1. Using the funnel, transfer the apple cider vinegar, witch hazel, and distilled water to the bottle. Discard excess.

2. Shake well.

how to use Using the spray bottle or a cotton ball, apply toner all over freshly cleansed face and neck.

tip This toner can be used on a cotton ball and applied only to extra-oily areas—for most people, this is their T-zone.

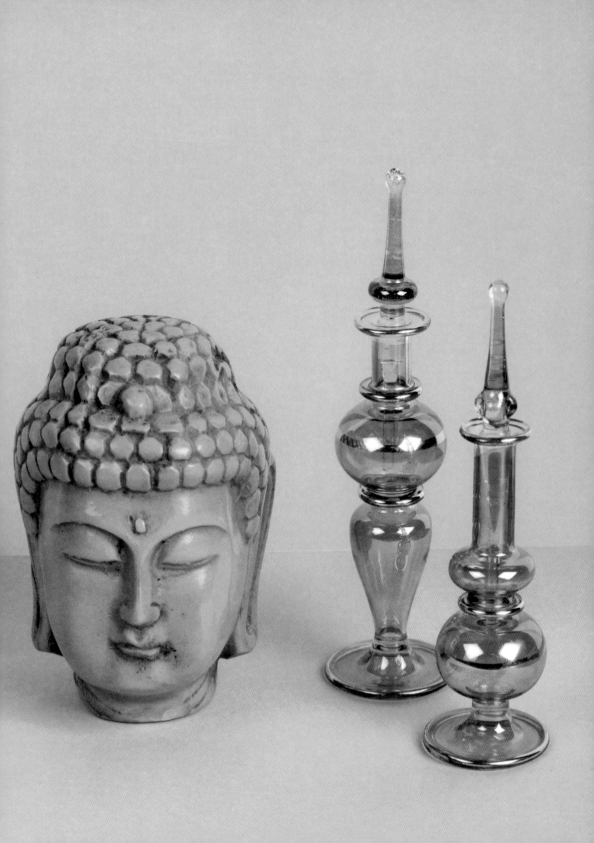

about the authors

Sisterpreneurs™ Caroline Bercaw and Isabel Bercaw are best known for cofounding a multimillion-dollar bath and body products company called Da Bomb Bath®. Over the past few years, their faces have graced the cover of *Entrepreneur Magazine* and they were included in the *Forbes* "30 Under 30 Class of 2019." All of this while juggling high school, friends, and running their company! But did you know they also have a passion for DIY makeup?

Growing up, the teens would spend countless hours playing with eye shadows, trying on different shades of lipstick, and admiring their mom's collection of blushes. Naturally, this translated into a hobby of creating makeup recipes of their own. (They're even planning to expand their current line of products to include some beauty-related offerings.) So, when they were given the opportunity to write a book all about natural beauty products, they couldn't refuse!

According to Caroline and Isabel, it's easy to make bath and beauty products at home without using synthetic additives or chemical preservatives. Their philosophy of simplicity is apparent in their first book, *Fizz Boom Bath!*, which features recipes for bath bombs and other fun bath and body treats, and has sold tens of thousands of copies all over the world. Now they're thrilled to present you with their latest creative effort, *Good Clean Beauty*. If you also love the idea of making your own eye shadows, body treatments, and more, this book is for you!

acknowledgments

We simply can't imagine a more exciting topic for our second book than DIY beauty. I mean, we've pretty much been preparing for this moment all our lives. Now that these pages are ready to go to press, some massive "thank-yous" are in order!

First of all, we'd like to offer our sincere gratitude to Publisher Rage Kindelsperger and Senior Editor John Foster for giving us the opportunity to participate in such a fun project. Rage is our ever-faithful champion and adviser for all things book-related, and we would be lost without her. John's impressive organizational talents, flexibility, and supportiveness were keys to the success of *Good Clean Beauty*. (P.S. He really knows how to defuse a panic attack!)

Next, a big, fantastic, hug-filled thank-you to Kiki Ely, whose radiant personality, mood-lifting attitude, and detailed knowledge of all things beauty really made this manuscript sing.

Another key factor in creating this book was our good fortune to work with a team that nailed the photography and art direction. Thank you so much to Creative Director Laura Drew, Photographer Liza Gershman, and Designer Laura Shaw for your truly impressive efforts.

Last but not least, we would like to thank our employees. They work tirelessly to help us grow our company and they support our various side hustles. They have always fueled our love for entrepreneurship and taught us a thing or two about friendship. We have also received endless support from our family, including our parents, Ben and Kim, and our grandparents, Barb, Ron, Mavis, and Bob. They're always excited to share our story with friends, relatives, and members of the general population, and we cannot thank you all enough for your continued enthusiasm.

index

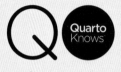

Brimming with creative inspiration, how-to projects, and useful information to enrich your everyday life, Quarto Knows is a favorite destination for those pursuing their interests and passions. Visit our site and dig deeper with our books into your area of interest: Quarto Creates, Quarto Cooks, Quarto Homes, Quarto Lives, Quarto Drives, Quarto Explores, Quarto Gifts, or Quarto Kids.

First published in 2020 by Rock Point,
an imprint of The Quarto Group
142 West 36th Street, 4th Floor
New York, NY 10018, USA
T (212) 779-4972 F (212) 779-6058
www.QuartoKnows.com

Rock Point titles are also available at discount for retail, wholesale, promotional, and bulk purchase. For details, contact the Special Sales Manager by email at specialsales@quarto.com or by mail at The Quarto Group, Attn: Special Sales Manager, 100 Cummings Center Suite 265D, Beverly, MA 01915 USA.

10 9 8 7 6 5 4 3 2 1

ISBN: 978-1-63106-659-7

Library of Congress Control Number: 2019952037

Recipe Development by Kiki Ely (Instagram: blonderambitions)
Photography by Liza Gershman
Photography on pages 6–15 © Shutterstock

Publisher: Rage Kindelsperger
Creative Director: Laura Drew
Managing Editor: Cara Donaldson
Senior Editor: John Foster
Cover and Interior Design: Laura Shaw

Printed in China

This book provides general information on various widely known and widely accepted images that tend to evoke feelings of strength and confidence. However, it should not be relied upon as recommending or promoting any specific diagnosis or method of treatment for a particular condition, and it is not intended as a substitute for medical advice or for direct diagnosis and treatment of a medical condition by a qualified physician. Readers who have questions about a particular condition, possible treatments for that condition, or possible reactions from the condition or its treatment should consult a physician or other qualified healthcare professional.